Dedication

To my mother, Susan, and father, Francis, who taught me at a very young age the importance of honesty, integrity, and respect for my fellow man, and to my mother-in-law, Florence Baron, who practiced these principles every day of her 81 years.

Esthetic Restorations:
Improved Dentist-Laboratory Communication

Paul J. Muia, BS, CDT
St Petersburg, Florida

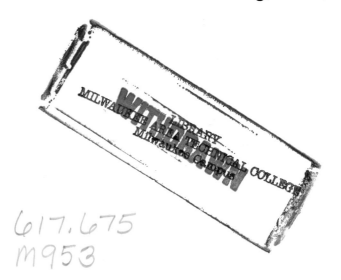

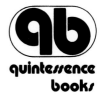

quinte**ss**ence
book**s**

Quintessence Publishing Co, Inc
Chicago, Berlin, London, Tokyo, São Paulo, and Moscow

"Knowledge advances by steps, not by leaps."
— *Thomas Bakinton MaCaulay (1800–1895)*

Library of Congress Cataloging-in-Publication Data

Muia, Paul J.
    Esthetic restorations : improved dentist-laboratory communication
/ Paul J. Muia.
        p.   cm.
    Includes index.
    ISBN 0-86715-226-5
    1. Fillings (Dentistry)   2. Dental ceramics.   3. Inlays
(Dentistry)   4. Dentistry—Esthetics.   5. Communication in
dentistry.   I. Title.
    [DNLM: 1. Dental Materials.   2. Dental Restoration, Permanent.
3. Esthetics, Dental.   WU 100 M953e 1993]
RK519.P65M85   1993
617.6'75—dc20
DNLM/DLC
for Library of Congress   92-48524
                                                                    CIP

© 1993 by Quintessence Publishing Co, Inc, Carol Stream, Illinois.
All rights reserved.

Editor: Laura G. Peppers
Design and Production: Timothy M. Robbins

Composition: Midwest Technical Publications, St Louis, MO
Printing and binding: Toppan Printing Co (S) Pte, Ltd, Singapore
Printed in Singapore

Contents

Foreword

Good communication between dentists and technicians has always presented a problem, particularly where there is no in-house laboratory. In his 35 years of laboratory experience, Paul Muia has had the fortune of working with some of the best clinicians in the USA. He is, therefore, well placed to pass on his knowledge to colleagues who may not have the opportunity to work closely with their clinicians, having instead to rely on information sent by post.

Success in clinical dentistry not only requires the patient to be happy with the esthetics and comfort of a restoration, but also requires its long-term survival. Paul Muia stresses the importance of correct metal-framework design to prevent fracture of the porcelain veneers and explains the difficulty of repairing porcelain in the event of fracture.

The mastery of the art and science of color communication is also emphasized, and Paul rightly stresses the need for technicians to make their own shade guides. This is well illustrated in his outstanding contribution known as "The Four Dimensional Tooth Color System." He refreshes our knowledge with further contributions on this subject and illustrates his expertise with detailed descriptions of how he constructs his clinical cases. In particular, his thoughts on dealing with the opaque layer reveal a deep understanding of the problem of avoiding high reflectivity from the metal surface, and his term "transition layer" aptly describes his efforts to increase the depth of translucency of his veneer porcelains.

The production of books on dental technology requires the dedication and discipline to fit photography sessions between the demands of routine laboratory work and the role of an author. Paul Muia is amongst the select few dental technicians who have achieved this and maintained the enthusiasm to set his thoughts down in print.

John W. McLean, OBE, FDS, RCS(Eng), DSc, MDS, Dr Odont

Preface

Over the past 35 years there have been many improvements in dental materials, techniques, and equipment. These accomplishments, although encouraging, are greatly overshadowed by the insignificant strides our profession has made in bringing the dentist and technician closer together as a *team*. Excellence in dentistry requires flawless dentist-technician communication, and only when working together as a team can this be accomplished.

In this book, my aim is to show the basic ingredients needed for a successful restoration and how the dentist and technician can work together so that these ingredients can be used to produce the best possible results. I have endeavored to make the dentist and technician more aware of what each must contend with in solving some of the clinical and technical problems that arise on a daily basis.

Currently, dentistry is attempting to find a replacement for the metal substructure in ceramic restorations. More all-ceramic restorations are being made, and there is no doubt that the 1990s will show great strides in this area. For a replacement material to metal to be acceptable, it must be strong enough to support a multiunit ceramic restoration with accuracy and vitality that will enhance the lifelike ceramic that covers it. It must be a material that resembles natural tooth structure chemically and physically and one that absorbs and reflects light in much the same way. There are some materials on the market today that have attempted to reach these goals; a few show promise but none have been completely successful.

However, until a material with the above qualities and the strength to support at least a six-unit splint is developed, we must rely on metal for ceramic substructure.

This book therefore describes ways to overcome some of the esthetic problems caused by metal substructure, while still taking advantage of its strength and accuracy. Every case should be well planned. Clinical and technical aspects should be thoroughly analyzed with input from both the dentist and technician. Chapter 1 thus focuses on the functional and esthetic needs for any given restoration and how a well-organized treatment plan ensures success.

After thorough planning, the fabrication begins with the metal substructure. Without an adequate foundation, the restoration cannot survive, regardless of its esthetic qualities. Chapter 2 covers aspects of the metal substructure, including alloy selection, substructure design, and proper waxing and casting techniques that will produce sufficient support for porcelain.

The next step in fabricating a restoration is color selection. Chapter 3 describes the four dimensions of color and the role each plays in natural dentition. Tooth color detection, measurement, and duplication are discussed, as is the customized tooth color guide.

To duplicate natural dentition exactly, knowledge of tooth irregularities is essential. Chapter 4 locates these irregularities and shows how each is incorporated into the restoration while duplicating the four tooth color dimensions.

Porcelain fractures are costly to both the dentist

and laboratory. Chapter 5 classifies porcelain fractures into three basic types and shows how each is prevented and repaired.

Finally, chapter 6 is a handy compendium of documented cases using information presented in the five previous chapters to show the importance of dentist-technician communication when attempting to fabricate an acceptable ceramic restoration.

This book is intended for all dentists, technicians and auxiliaries regardless of experience or educational background. I have included information that will especially be of use to the entire dental team. Although my 35 year career in dentistry has been spent in an in-office laboratory environment, I have presented this information in a way that dentist-technician communication in a separated environment can benefit as well.

Chapter 1

Case Planning

Success or failure of a dental restoration depends greatly on how well critical information is communicated between dentist and laboratory. It is the dentist's responsibility to accurately evaluate the function, contour, and color for each case, and further, to formulate a means of communicating this information to the laboratory that will ensure completion of an acceptable restoration.

At least 75% of all remakes are caused by poor communication. The frustration and embarrassment, plus the loss of time, profits, and credibility, are suffered by both the dentist and laboratory technician. A strained relationship often results and, sometimes, a complete.severing of the business relationship. Therefore, every restoration, regardless how extensive, should begin with case planning. After a preliminary examination, the dentist thoroughly describes the intended treatment plan to the patient. A discussion should then cover certain basic information and choices.

First, the patient's oral health should be evaluated, including periodontal and bone health. Mounted diagnostic maxillary and mandibular models should show occlusion and what can be done to improve any unhealthy conditions that are present; visual aids of these areas are helpful during discussion with the patient (Figs 1-1a to c). They permit the dentist to show and discuss ideal dental health and compare it with that of the patient. They also give the patient a better understanding of how the dentist hopes to improve these conditions and make it easier for the patient to make a decision should the opportunity present itself. Above all, a clear, simple discussion builds confidence between patient and dentist. Any additional evaluations by an endodontist, periodontist, orthodontist, or oral surgeon should be conducted before initiating the proposed treatment plan.

After the initial evaluation, the dentist discusses the proposed treatment plan and calls on the laboratory for any technical advice that may help him or her decide the most appropriate materials and techniques for a particular case. Whenever necessary, case planning should include the dentist, patient, and technician. The dentist must determine the needs for each patient and certainly make the final decisions; however, input by the technician as to feasible techniques and materials should be considered before the decisions are finalized.

All comments made by the patient should be made part of his or her record. When in doubt as to the technical possibilities, the dentist should confer with the laboratory before assuring the patient that certain requests can be fulfilled. Only then is it possible to predict how the patient will react toward the completed restoration.

Case planning information that must be sent to the laboratory should be placed in four categories, in order of importance: (1) function, (2) contour, (3) color, and (4) patient's comments. These areas will be discussed in detail.

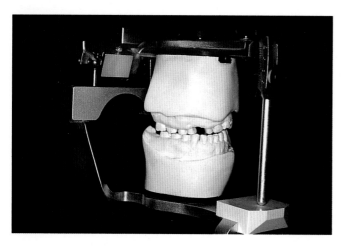

Fig 1-1a Mounted diagnostic models are not only essential for case evaluation by the dentist, they should also be used as a guide for the laboratory. A model helps in explaining to the patient the proposed treatment plan and helps in discussing with the technician possible procedures and materials that will be used to comply with that treatment. Duplicate models are used for fabricating the provisional restoration.

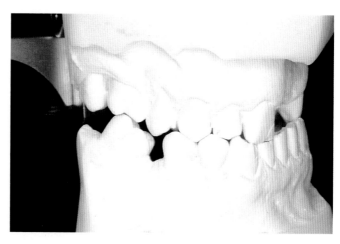

Fig 1-1b A close-up view showing tooth shifting brought about by poor dental maintenance. With a diagnostic model, problem areas can be isolated and discussed separately, while establishing an appropriate treatment plan that will satisfy everyone involved.

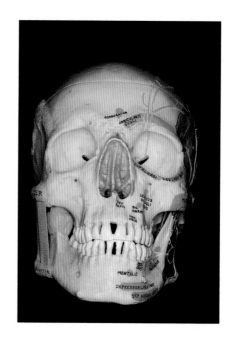

Fig 1-1c Visual aids are used by many dentists to show the patient the healthy and unhealthy conditions found in the mouth. They not only help the dentist describe to the patient needed treatment but in most cases create an incentive for the patient to improve dental care.

Function

Function supercedes all esthetic considerations (ie, contour and color). A single unit can affect function; the more units involved, the more complicated the treatment becomes and the greater the role function plays in dictating the approach to this treatment.

Both the dentist and technician must be aware of the clinical and technical needs of each case. These functional needs should be placed in certain categories and itemized so that the technician can perfectly understand the intent of the dentist. Information conveyed by the dentist should include: (1) preferred occlusion principles; (2) preferred alloy for metal substructure; (3) preferred material for occlusal surfaces; (4) mounted models; (5) anterior guide table; (6) preferred material for margins (porcelain or metal); and (7) comments concerning potential problems.

Preferred Occlusion Principles

Most dentists are consistent in their preference of occlusion principle. It is important, however, to evaluate each case in order to determine which principle is most appropriate.

Tripodization

The gnathologic approach to occlusion uses tripodization as a means to a mesiodistal stabilization of posterior teeth in the long axis. The cusps of posterior teeth make contact with the sides of the fossa of the opposite teeth in centric occlusion. It is believed that support such as this eliminates the need for splinting weakly supported teeth. This theory is enforced by the fact that every cusp has four ridges. Three of the four ridges can contact an opposing cusp (tripodization) and form a Gothic pyramid. Therefore, two rounded surfaces meet at a point so the contacts will be small, and this should promote a built-in adjustability to wear.

Before selecting tripodization as the basic functional aspect for the case, the dentist considers the condition of the opposing dentition and whether or not it will be restored. Ideal cusp formation and position should be present or restored so as to promote proper occlusion. Demands for perfect conditions are high with tripodization, and if these conditions are not present, other occlusal methods must be explored.

Cusp Tip-to-Fossa

A somewhat less critical type of occlusion and an alternative to tripodization is the cusp tip-to-fossa theory. Function and stability are achieved when cusp tips are properly located. Cusp tip location is flexible and can be designed to suit the case. The condition of opposing dentition is not as critical as in tripodization. Cusp tips can be properly located with less concern for opposing cusp contour and location, making cusp tip-to-fossa an ideal selection for cases where opposing dentition is not appropriate for tripodization. The cusp tip contacts the opposing fossa, making a definite stop. It is not necessary to restore the maxillary and mandibular arch together, thus making for more flexibility.

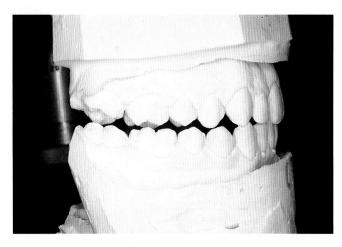

Fig 1-2 Articulated maxillary and mandibular models in the left lateral excursion showing posterior disocclusion, gliding over the lingual surface of the right canine. Posterior disocclusion is prescribed only when the canines have adequate periodontal support.

Canine-Protected (Posterior) Disocclusion (Fig 1-2)

Under normal conditions, the maxillary canines are the strongest and best supported teeth in the mouth. They are often called upon to disocclude premolars and molars during lateral excursions. Regardless which teeth are involved in the restoration, if the dentist thinks the posterior teeth should be protected and the canines are healthy enough to carry the load, the laboratory staff must be so informed. If the posterior teeth are being restored, care must be taken to contour the buccal aspects so that during lateral excursion they disocclude immediately and completely and are out of contact with opposing cusps. This can be accomplished with either cusp-to-fossa or cusp tip-to-fossa type occlusion. If the dentist thinks the canine is not able to take the entire load, other steps should be taken to alleviate the problem.

Group Function (Figs 1-3a and b)

"Group function" is a method used successfully in cases where the dentist feels the canines cannot carry the entire load during lateral excursion. In group function, during excursions, the load is distributed evenly over several or all posterior teeth. The dentist must instruct the technician which posterior teeth should be in contact during lateral excursion and whether contact should be unilateral or bilateral.

In porcelain veneer restorations associated with group function, the metal substructure must be designed to give maximum support to the porcelain. If the metal substructure is not extended to support the added length of porcelain, fracture could occur causing failure. The added trauma of removing the restoration due to failure could further damage the teeth involved in the treatment plan.

Failure on the part of the dentist or technician to heed the necessity for group function on a particular case could cause further deterioration of already unhealthy bone structure, with the possibility of eventual tooth loss.

Anterior Centric Stops (Fig 1-4)

When maxillary and mandibular anterior teeth are involved in the treatment plan, the dentist must decide whether or not centric stops or contacts with opposing dentition are needed. Mounted diagnostic models will be helpful in determining this. However, a thorough evaluation should be made, noting especially the effect the tongue and lips have in preventing the anterior teeth from supraeruption. When anterior teeth are splinted, there is less chance of supraeruption; however, individually restored teeth with no centric stops or tongue and lip support could supraerupt.

The dentist must also consider phonetic involvement. To achieve anterior centric stops with individually restored teeth, added length may be required. In complicated cases where both

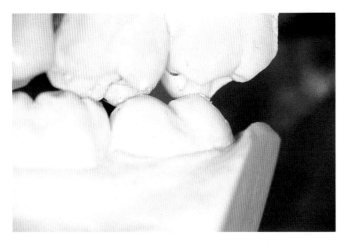

Fig 1-3a Articulated case in left lateral excursion, showing lingual cusps of maxillary left first and second molars in contact with buccal cusps of the mandibular first and second molars. The molars, in this case, will share some of the load that would otherwise be the responsibility of the maxillary right canine.

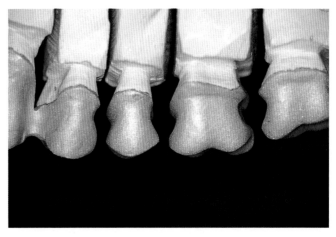

Fig 1-3b Properly contoured metal substructure for a restoration involving group function during right and left lateral excursions. Group function usually requires extended porcelain cusp tips on the restoration so that a smooth, well-organized slide will occur during excursions. To prevent a porcelain fracture in these areas, the metal substructure must be contoured to support the extended cusp tips. Also, note the connection between the canine and first premolar; it lends added support to the canine. This, along with group function, will share the load during lateral excursion.

maxillary and mandibular arches are being restored, proper contour and length for centric stops are essential, making it imperative that the laboratory be instructed accordingly.

It is impossible to establish strict rules governing occlusion. The above occlusal concepts are perhaps the most important ones to be considered of the many that make up the complicated gnathostomatic system. The articulating surfaces, with the muscles and ligaments, make up this system, and disharmony brought about by insufficient dentist-technician communication could result in dysfunction and cause further deterioration.

Preferred Alloy for Metal Substructure

A factor often overlooked is the alloy selection for the metal substructures. The dentist carefully eval-

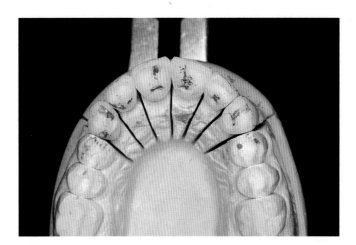

Fig 1-4 Lingual surface of maxillary anterior restorations, revealing centric stops and glide paths taken during lateral excursions and protrusive movement. Note position of centric stops. They should never be located on an incline or a convexity; each should have a definite seat to prevent tooth movement when units are not connected.

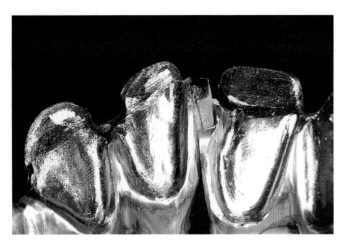

Fig 1-5 Multiunit metal substructure, tied together with a dovetail. The dentist and/or laboratory technician should foresee potential problems associated with the metal substructure when selecting the alloy for the case. In cases such as this, metal hardness is a necessity.

uates which alloy is best suited for the case, keeping in mind that if the metal does not meet the requirements the restoration could fail. The laboratory should have an assortment of several alloys that can meet the needs of any given case (see Chapter 2). The available choices should range from a relatively high-gold-content alloy to hard base metal alloy. Selection is based on needed strength and hardness, periodontal involvement, restoration location, and any other prerequisite for a successful restoration. The dentist must be able to foresee any potential problem that could arise because of improper alloy selection and further should prescribe the alloy that will best prevent the problem. For example, a much stronger and harder base metal alloy should be considered over a softer noble metal alloy in splints that need great strength in thin interproximal areas or in splints that must resist wear. On the other hand, cases that require a "cushion" effect because of periodontal involvement or in patients where resistance to wear is a concern, a high-gold-content noble metal alloy might be considered (Fig 1-5).

Preferred Material for Occluding Surface

A decision must also be made as to the most appropriate material for the occluding surface of the restoration. Materials for occluding surfaces can be classified as (1) porcelain, (2) metal, and (3) porcelain-metal combination. As in metal substructures, selection should be made according to several factors and will vary from case to case. Periodontal involvement and opposing dentition must be taken into consideration in order to make the proper decision based on material hardness and wear resistance.

Material hardness ranges from a relatively soft high-gold-content alloy to very hard base metal alloy, with porcelain ranking somewhere between the two.

Porcelain Occluding Surface

To many patients, porcelain is the most esthetic material because it resembles natural dentition. For this reason, when patients are given a choice, they usually select porcelain over metal or a combination of the two. Most patients prefer that no metal be visible in the restoration, hence the entire occlusal surface must be covered with porcelain. Under normal conditions therefore, porcelain is usually the material selected for occluding surfaces.

There are cases, however, where porcelain may not be the best selection. Porcelain, being somewhat harder than noble metal alloys, will not be the choice of the dentist who prefers to accept the "cushion effect" theory. This theory states that the harder the occluding material, the greater the chance of damaging the periodontal tissue, and it holds true especially in cases where periodontal problems are found to exist prior to restoration. When examining a patient who has porcelain occluding with a high-gold-content noble metal alloy restoration, it is not uncommon to see wear patterns worn into the metal by porcelain, which shows no sign of wear. This is particularly found with unglazed porcelain. The resiliency of the gold and its low resistance to wear lends to the theory that gold does indeed contribute to preserving the health of the tissue and bone surrounding the teeth. Even though a properly equilibrated maxillary and mandibular arch will minimize the amount of wear to opposing dentition, it is worth recognizing that although porcelain occluding surfaces are by far the most esthetic, their hardness and resistance to wear could in some cases be a contributing factor to periodontal problems.

The feasibility of porcelain occluding surfaces should be determined during case planning. If the dentist finds that after considering all the consequences it will not further deteriorate the present dental health of the patient, porcelain occlusal surfaces should be prescribed. When in doubt as to its feasibility, other possibilities should be explored.

Metal Occluding Surfaces

There are several reasons for selecting metal occluding surfaces: (1) to create a "cushion effect," (2) to prevent wear to opposing dentition, (3) when there is insufficient room for porcelain coverage, and (4) for critical occlusal accuracy.

Cushion effect. As previously noted, some dentists think that certain noble metal alloys (especially those with high-gold content) are less stressful to teeth and surrounding tissue and bone. Some dentists prefer a much softer full-gold casting for posterior teeth with no porcelain, rather than a noble metal alloy with porcelain, which is harder.

Going from high-gold-content noble metal alloy to a much harder base metal alloy, the gold content decreases and other elements are added. The metal becomes progressively harder and less effective in contributing to a cushion effect. When extra strength is needed in the metal substructure due to skimpy connections or ultrafine margin

bevels, a compromise must be made to satisfy both the cushion effect and the needed strength. This would mean selecting a noble metal alloy with slightly less gold content to increase strength hardness but yet soft enough to ensure less trauma to involved teeth.

Wear to opposing dentition. The same principle holds true to the effect on the opposing dentition; the softer the metal occluding surface (high-gold content), the less wear to the opposing dentition. As the gold content decreases, wear to the opposing dentition increases. It seems logical, therefore, that when tissue health and tooth wear is of concern, a noble alloy with a high-gold content should be selected.

Insufficient room for porcelain. Occasionally, a restoration displays insufficient room for porcelain, making it necessary to use a metal occluding surface for centric stops. The available room will help determine alloy selection. The higher the gold content, the more thickness is needed for required alloy strength. Necessary metal thickness varies from 0.3 mm in high-gold-content alloy to 0.1 mm in base metal alloys. In certain cases that require an ultrathin metal occluding surface, it may necessitate sacrificing the cushion effect derived from the soft, high-gold-content alloy and choosing a harder alloy with lower gold content, which supplies great strength in spite of ultrathinness.

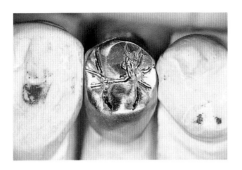

Fig 1-6a

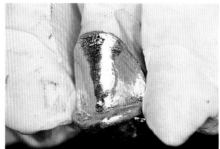

Fig 1-6b

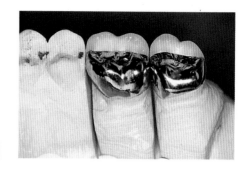

Fig 1-7

Fig 1-6a Maxillary premolar: noble alloy substructure with metal occlusal surface. This is the softest occlusal surface possible in a metal ceramic restoration. In this case, there is a need to take advantage of the "cushion effect" afforded by the noble alloy. Lack of necessary occlusal thickness, concern for occluding wear of opposing dentition, and need for metal occlusal surface are other reasons for selecting a soft metal (noble alloy) occlusal surface.

Fig 1-6b Buccal view of premolar showing area to be covered with porcelain. Note buccal occlusal ledge. It provides a porcelain finish line with protection from occlusal forces.

Fig 1-7 Two maxillary molars with porcelain-metal occlusal surfaces, satisfying the esthetic and functional needs of the restoration.

Critical occlusion accuracy (Figs 1-6a and b). It is important to attain accurate occlusion and function in every case. There are cases, however, that require more attention. Malocclusion, temporomandibular dysfunction, and bruxism are examples of cases that require even more accuracy and stability than normal cases that depend on porcelain occlusion. It is much easier to establish definite occlusal anatomy through waxing rather than by building in porcelain. Once the desired goals are established in wax, the finished casting will maintain them. It is more difficult to obtain the same results through porcelain fabrication due to porcelain shrinkage, required repeated firings, and having to grind in needed anatomy.

Where absolute accuracy in occlusion and function is a top priority, a metal casting that was precisely waxed surpasses that of a porcelain occluding surface and should be considered, even with the possible sacrifice of esthetics.

Porcelain-Metal Occluding Surface (Fig 1-7)

An alternative to an all-porcelain or all-metal occluding surface is a combination of both. By combining porcelain and metal for the occluding surface, it is possible to derive benefit from each.

Needless to say, the porcelain labial or buccal surface lends to the esthetics of the restoration, permitting the ceramist to duplicate natural tooth color and contour. The metal portion of the occluding surface will satisfy either or all of the following: (1) cushion effect (high-gold-content noble metal alloy), (2) strength for thin metal substructures (low-gold-content noble metal alloy or base metal alloy), and (3) critical cusp contacts and anterior centric stops (all alloys, from high-gold content to base metal).

Posteriorly, metal lingual cusps contribute to either the cushion effect or needed strength and critical cusp contacts. Anteriorly, metal lingual surfaces serving as centric stops satisfy the cushion effect, or supply the needed strength in ultrathin areas.

The material for the occluding surface should be selected during case planning. All functional and esthetic factors must be considered. Of the several possibilities, the one most advantageous to both function and esthetics is the porcelain-metal combination. It offers the opportunity to conceal most of the metal functional surfaces with porcelain, thus combining ultimate function with esthetics.

Mounted Models and Guidelines

All of the above information is classified as written or verbal communication. However, models and guidelines fall into the category of *visual communication*. Written and verbal communication give an overall description of the case, conveying to the laboratory staff basic functional and esthetic expectations. Perhaps even more important are the more tangible models and guidelines.

Mounted Diagnostic Models
(see Figs 1-1a and b)

Mounted diagnostic models show the laboratory technician the pretreatment condition of the patient's mouth. They not only help locate existing functional problems, they also alert both the dentist and technician to any potential posttreatment functional problems that could occur as a direct result of the seated permanent restoration. Practically the entire treatment plan can be established after examining the mounted diagnostic models, which can clearly point out functional defects ranging from a simple premature contact to a major malocclusion. These models also permit the dentist to point out to the patient existing problems, combining verbal explanation with a visual aid that will most certainly make the problems and the plan for treating these problems more clear.

Mounted Models of Seated Provisional Restoration

It may take several visits to "fine tune" the functional and esthetic aspects of the provisional restoration, because the patient must be given time to recognize any physical or functional problem that may be present and any unacceptable esthetic disharmony. When the dentist and patient feel the provisional restoration is functionally and esthetically acceptable, an impression is taken and a model made. The model should be mounted on the same articulator as the mounted diagnostic model so that it is interchangeable with it.

The mounted model of the provisional restoration, whether it be mandibular or maxillary, serves several purposes. It gives the dentist an opportunity to further explain to the patient the treatment plan by comparing the mounted diagnostic model with the mounted model of the provisional restoration. Contemplated improvements in function and esthetics can be more easily conveyed than with merely a verbal description. More importantly, the model gives the technician a guide throughout the entire fabrication of the restoration. Both models should be interchangeable with the master working model, thus giving the technician an opportunity to refer back to not only the present provisional restoration but also to the original pretreatment condition of the patient, should the need arise. The technician should carefully analyze the three mounted models before beginning construction and if he or she has any concerns about the feasibility of the treatment plan should immediately alert the dentist. Any potential problem or uncertainty must be resolved at this time, and often a phone call to the dentist is sufficient to prevent the fabrication of an otherwise unacceptable restoration.

The model of the seated provisional restoration serves other useful purposes. It is the source for the customized anterior guide table, anterior index, and the every-other-tooth model.

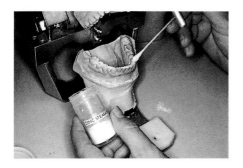

Fig 1-8a

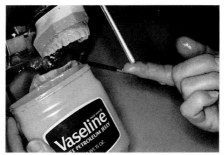

Fig 1-8b

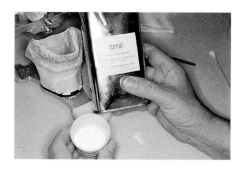

Fig 1-8c

Fig 1-8a   A powder, such as zinc stearate, is applied to the incisal edge and occlusal surface of the opposing mandibular arch to prevent wear during articulator manipulation while establishing anterior guide table. A fine talcum powder will serve the same purpose.

Fig 1-8b   A thin layer of petroleum jelly is applied to the tip of the guide pin so that it will glide freely over the acrylic resin, forming a smooth, accurate path. If not lubricated properly, the pin could stick to the acrylic resin and cause distortion and roughness during manipulation.

Fig 1-8c   Acrylic resin powder and liquid manufactured especially for the fabrication of the anterior guide table. If this is not available, any cold-cure acrylic resin can be used.

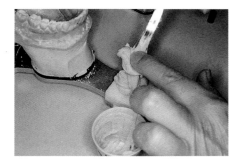

Fig 1-8d

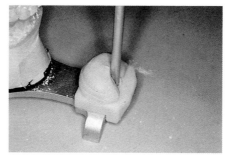

Fig 1-8e

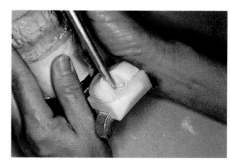

Fig 1-8f

Fig 1-8d   When the powder-liquid mixture reaches the doughy stage (workable, with no evidence of tackiness), it is placed on the table of the articulator and shaped into a mound.

Fig 1-8e   The articulator is closed, making sure the pin strikes its floor. It is important to establish a definite stop that corresponds to the centric stops on the lingual surface of the maxillary anterior teeth.

Fig 1-8f   The pin is moved to the extreme right, forming a glide path that represents right lateral excursion. The contour of this glide path is dictated primarily by the lingual surface of the maxillary left canine.

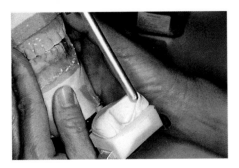

Fig 1-8g

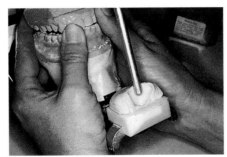

Fig 1-8h

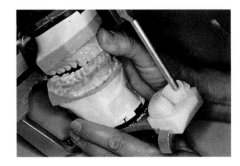

Fig 1-8i

Fig 1-8g   The pin is then moved to the extreme left, forming the glide path of the left lateral excursion, which is dictated by the lingual surface of the maxillary right canine.

Fig 1-8h   The articulator is placed into protrusive position by moving the guide pin posteriorly. This maneuver is mainly responsible for transferring the entire lingual contour of the four maxillary incisors along with the remaining contour of the canines, which was not registered during lateral excursions. The protrusive maneuver of the articulator also transfers the length of the four maxillary incisors onto the anterior guide table (the canine lengths are established during lateral excursions).

Fig 1-8i   Articulator in left lateral excursion, revealing posterior disocclusion. The canine length is a constant, derived by the functional and phonetic needs of the patient. The length of the maxillary buccal cusps, however, is variable and can be altered to either disocclude (ie, be shortened) or to work in group function (ie, be lengthened) during restoration of the posterior teeth.

Customized Anterior Guide Table (Figs 1-8a to i)

The customized anterior guide table is a duplication of the lingual contour of the maxillary six anterior teeth. This contour is derived from protrusive and lateral excursions and is precisely refined to accommodate the ideal relationship between the anterior maxillary and mandibular teeth. The customized anterior guide table can be patterned after the original diagnostic model of the maxillary arch before preparation. This would hold true in cases where the anterior mandibular teeth are being treated alone and before preparing the maxillary arch. These cases do not absolutely require a guide table, whether the opposing model is diagnostic or provisional, but it does ensure exact mandibular movements and prevents excessive wear to the maxillary model that could necessitate adjustment of the seated restoration.

The guide table is especially important when the anterior maxillary teeth are involved in the restoration. The lingual contour of these teeth is established in the restoration through the efforts of the guide table and should be included in the fabrication of the restoration before the waxing begins.

After mounting the master working model, the technician can evaluate the available lingual working room by manipulating the articulator in lateral and protrusive movements. This will immediately show not only the required length of the canines and possibly the four incisors, but also the eventual thickness of the lingual aspect of the restoration. This will help determine whether it is possible to have porcelain cover metal in this area. If indications show that this area does not afford enough room for both porcelain and metal, a metal strike or an entire metal lingual glide path may have to be introduced. This evaluation will also show if enough tooth reduction was made. This must be determined before waxing begins because, should the anterior maxillary teeth not clear the opposing mandibular teeth with enough room to allow for porcelain and metal, the guidance could be subsequently steepened, possibly resulting in TMJ dysfunction.

At this point, if the technician finds that tooth reduction has indeed been insufficient, the dentist must be notified and possible arrangements made to reduce the die or dies on the master working model. The dentist can alter the dies to a dimension that is functionally acceptable. A "cutoff" coping is constructed for the dentist to use as a guide for trimming the prepared tooth or teeth before attempting to place the restoration. A casting is made of the wax pattern of the recontoured die.

After all the requirements in regard to the guide table are satisfied at the prewaxing stage, the case can proceed to the waxing stage.

Waxing Stage

During the waxing stage, the anterior guide table will dictate the lingual contour of the six maxillary anterior teeth. Waxing should be taken to full contour, and upon completion, the lingual aspect of the wax pattern is refined with the guide table if that surface is to be metal. Should it be designated for porcelain, an even thickness of wax is removed in conjunction with the labial reduction. Lingual porcelain should not exceed 1 mm and must be uniform throughout. After cutting back the wax over the entire pattern, the guide table is engaged in lateral excursions and protrusive movement to verify adequate room for porcelain. Protrusive movement will also ensure proper length and incisal thickness.

When the wax pattern can be moved freely through all excursions over the path supplied by the guide table, the case can be prepared for casting. After casting and metal finishing, the frame is ready for porcelain fabrication.

Porcelain Fabrication

When the lingual surface of the restoration is to be metal, the lateral and protrusive movements will have been established during the waxing stage. When the lingual surface is to be porcelain, however, the entire porcelain fabrication, pre- and postfiring, will depend entirely on the guide table.

In the porcelain buildup stage, care must be taken during excursions not to disturb the prefired porcelain. The slightest particle disarrangement could cause microscopic separation that after firing will cause weakness in the restoration with probable future fracture. More serious disturbances will bring about visible fissures and immediate fracture to the fired porcelain. During preglaze shaping, care must be taken to follow the guide table precisely. As with the lingual contour of the six maxillary teeth, canine length and glide path must be duplicates of the diagnostic or provisional model so that they will function as prescribed by the dentist (ie, complete posterior disocclusion or full or partial group function). Its ability or inability to support the complete load during lateral excursions will dictate the role it will play.

Of all the tangible guidelines the dentist could communicate to the laboratory technician, perhaps the one with the most functional significance is the anterior guide table. It establishes the exact movements the mandible must make to provide the patient with optimum function and comfort. The technician cannot accomplish this without the guide table.

Preferred Margin: Metal or Porcelain

Metal Labial or Buccal Margins

Until the advent of labial porcelain margins, metal margins prevailed exclusively. Acceptable esthetics and gingival health are directly proportional to tooth preparation and how well the metal margin can be covered with porcelain. In order to properly cover the opaqued metal margin to satisfy esthetics and gingival health, the preparation has to have enough tooth structure removed to allow for a porcelain thickness that will completely cover the metal margin yet be thin enough not to impinge on the tissue. In many instances this is difficult to accomplish, especially in cases that prohibit adequate tooth reduction. Gingival irritation and recession result from bulky porcelain at the labial or buccal margin. Although many gingival problems are eliminated with properly contoured gingival areas, and even though the metal margin is well covered, a shadow is often visible. Most patients notice this immediately and some will be dissatisfied.

Porcelain Labial or Buccal Margins

An alternative to the metal margin is the porcelain margin. With a porcelain margin, the gingival third of the restoration can be more easily contoured to conform with the gingival boundaries, thus eliminating the possibility of impingement with eventual recession. Porcelain margins also avoid the shadow often associated with a metal margin. A well-glazed porcelain surface is kinder to the gingiva than other dental material. Therefore, a restoration with porcelain margins in most cases will show better tissue response than one with metal margins and is highly recommended where superior tissue response is a necessity. When possible, and especially in the anterior region, porcelain margins should be considered.

During case planning, the dentist should present the patient with both possibilities, pointing out the advantages of each. If feasible, the patient should be given the opportunity to choose the type of margin that will best suit his or her needs and expectations.

There are several techniques to choose from when incorporating porcelain margins in a ceramic restoration. The three methods most widely used today are: (1) building body porcelain directly to the shoulder of the die, (2) building body porcelain to a platinum matrix, and (3) building body porcelain to a previously formed margin derived from a special margin material.

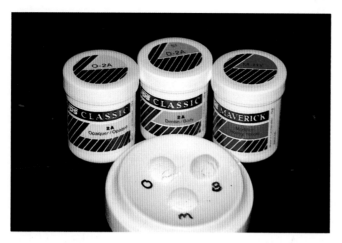

Fig 1-9a Three components that make up the transition layer (O-B-M): (1) Opaque: The prescribed opaque for the selected hue-chroma dimension (dentin). (2) Body: The body porcelain selected for the dentin build-up (hue). Should the chroma dimension (diluted version of the hue) be selected for the body build-up, the portion is measured after the dilution has been accomplished. (3) Maverick: The maverick dimension selected to complete the CTC. If a premixed maverick color is not available, a body modifier with proper amount of neutral porcelain can be used.

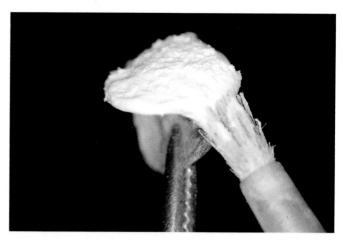

Fig 1-9b Applying transition layer to casting. The transition layer covers the opaque layer completely and is fired before attempting to establish the porcelain margin. The surface of this layer is always made rough to diffuse light and reflect color.

Body porcelain to die shoulder (Figs 1-9a to d). In this method for constructing porcelain margins, body porcelain is applied directly to the shoulder of the die during porcelain buildup. As in all procelain margin cases, the tooth preparation must resemble that of a porcelain jacket crown in the area designated for a porcelain margin. A 90-degree angle with no bevel should be evident.

The stone die must be prepared to accept wet body porcelain. This is usually accomplished in two steps. First, sealant liquid is applied to the shoulder of the die to seal the pores of the stone, thus preventing the possibility of liquid loss from the wet porcelain due to absorption. It may take several applications to ensure a thorough seal. Second, when the sealant is completely dry, and immediately before porcelain application, a releasing agent is applied to the shoulder.

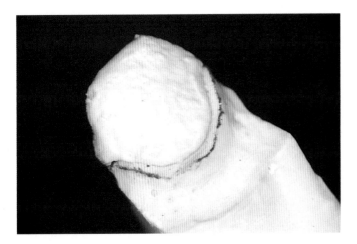

Fig 1-9c The fired transition layer is placed onto the die after the die has been thoroughly sealed. The shoulder of the prepared tooth should be as close as possible to a 90-degree angle. Any angle other than this will tend to cause the porcelain to pull away from the shoulder of the die. Also, if the angle is more than 90 degrees, a "gray margin" is likely to develop, caused by thin, translucent porcelain in this area. To prevent a gray margin, a thin application of transition porcelain can be applied to the shoulder immediately before building body porcelain to it. Both applications are fired simultaneously.

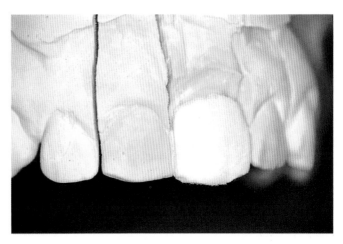

Fig 1-9d Prefired body and enamel porcelain that has been applied directly to the sealed shoulder of the die. These layers can be applied and fired individually or together. When using this method to obtain porcelain margins, the latter is suggested. A well-condensed porcelain buildup will ensure minimum shrinkage at the margin. Some shrinkage will occur, however, and this can be resolved to some extent during the glaze firing. A mixture of transition and body porcelain (1:2) is applied to the margin and placed onto the die. Once the void has been filled, the restoration is fired under vacuum to approximately 10 degrees below maturing temperature, then hand polished to obtain the desired glaze.

Body porcelain is applied before the releasing agent dries and is condensed well. The more condensing, the less shrinkage in this area and the better the sealed margin. After porcelain buildup, the restoration is fired. Regardless of how well the porcelain is condensed, some shrinkage will occur. Several firings of porcelain additions must be made in order to achieve an acceptable marginal seal.

Of the three methods for constructing a porcelain margin, this is the least desirable because regardless of how many firings are performed, there is always some shrinkage with a certain amount of porcelain "roll back." This means there is never a perfect marginal seal. Therefore, when using this method, it is virtually impossible to obtain a seal as efficient as that obtained using the other two methods to be discussed.

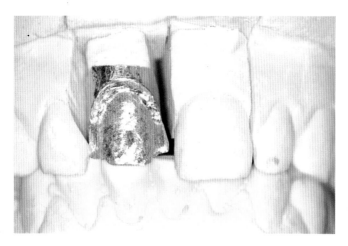

Fig 1-10a Platinum matrix with casting. A well-adapted matrix over the labial or buccal shoulder will produce a well-sealed porcelain margin with no extra firings. (The platinum should be annealed before burnishing.) The platinum must prevent the casting from seating uniformly around the entire circumference of the die so that when removing it upon completing the restoration, a perfect seal will occur.

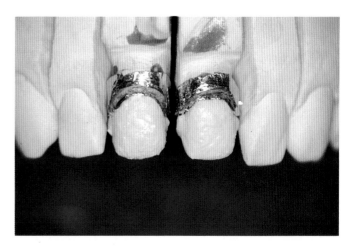

Fig 1-10b Fired transition layer holding platinum matrix in place. At this stage the platinum is attached to the casting and is ready for final burnishing before body buildup. In this method the porcelain margin is developed with a separate "donut bake" (body porcelain is overbuilt in the margin area and fired). Porcelain will shrink toward the margin and create a perfect seal. Dentin and enamel layers are then applied and fired. After contouring and glazing, the platinum is removed and the restorations are ready for seating.

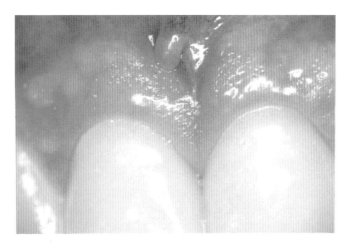

Fig 1-10c Seated maxillary central incisors (from Fig 1-10b) after 3-day recall showing how well the tissue has adapted to the porcelain margins. When properly executed, the platinum method for obtaining a porcelain margin will produce a sharp finish line with an excellent marginal seal.

Body porcelain to platinum matrix (Figs 1-10a to c). A method designed to produce a more acceptable marginal seal involves a platinum matrix at the labial or buccal shoulder of the die. Platinum (0.001 mm) is adapted to the die and extended 2 mm onto the labial surface while maintaining an apron of equal length over the shoulder. The casting, with a fired opaque wash, is placed over the degassed platinum matrix while being attached with several small drops of cyanoacrylate adhesive. After the platinum is burnished to the die, the casting is covered with a transition layer (opaque, body and maverick) and carried far enough to just contact the matrix. The casting with attached matrix is carefully removed from the die and fired. The matrix is now part of the casting, held together with the transition layer.

After placing the casting back on the die, the platinum is burnished well to the shoulder of the

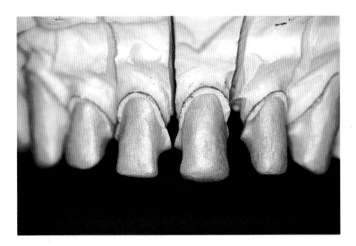

Fig 1-11a Castings on dies that have been specially prepared to accept a porcelain margin. The closer to a 90-degree shoulder preparation, the better chance of a perfect marginal seal. The shoulders of the dies are coated with a liquid sealant, which upon drying will prevent the absorption of liquid from the porcelain mixture. This can be applied while the castings are being opaqued. The sealant liquid is usually supplied with the porcelain margin material kit.

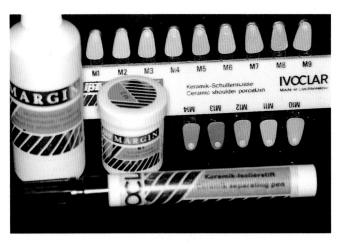

Fig 1-11b A porcelain system designed specifically for incorporating a labial porcelain margin into a restoration (Ivoclar-Williams). This is the most popular method for developing porcelain margins. A complete kit should include a sealant, releasant, special build-up liquid, and a wide range of colors and modifiers along with a color guide to help make appropriate selections. A perfect marginal seal is imperative, therefore the manufacturer's instructions must be followed precisely.

die and porcelain is applied to it. The porcelain is overbuilt on the matrix and slightly feathered onto the casting. This is fired separately so that the shrinkage takes place toward the shoulder; porcelain shrinks to the area of greatest bulk. The fired casting is placed back on the die and is prepared for the body buildup, which should include all the color dimensions along with any needed characterizations. After final contour and glaze, the platinum matrix is removed.

When properly adapted, the platinum matrix should prevent the crown from seating on the die. The degree of opening should be uniform throughout the entire circumference of the restoration so that upon removal of the matrix, the finished restoration will seat perfectly with a superior seal.

Body porcelain to preformed porcelain margin (Figs 1-11a to c). Most ceramists currently use a special porcelain compound designed especially for constructing a porcelain margin. The material is used to fabricate the margin upon completion of the opaque layer. It is applied directly to the shoulder of the die, which has been treated with a sealant and releasant, and is extended on the opaqued casting to about 1.5 mm. The material must be vibrated well and slightly overbuilt. There is usually slight shrinkage upon firing, thus a second application and firing are required. After contouring and cleansing, the opaqued casting with its preformed margin is ready for porcelain application.

The basic principle behind this method is the maturing temperature difference between the four

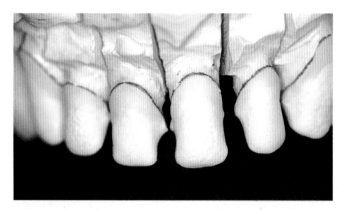

Fig 1-11c Second firing of porcelain margin material. Two applications of margin material are usually required for a complete seal. Each application requires a releasing agent to be painted over the shoulder area so that the porcelain can be easily removed from the die. The porcelain is now ready to be chamfered and prepared for the application of the transition layer, over which will be fired the dentin and enamel layers. Firing temperatures are progressively lower for each stage.

mediums: opaque, margin material, transition layer, and body porcelain. The opaque and body porcelain have the highest and lowest maturing temperatures respectively, of the four, whereas the margin material has a maturing temperature between the two. Thus, the opaque layer is undisturbed during the processing of the margin material, which is undisturbed during the porcelain fabrication.

This method for producing porcelain margins has a high percentage of success, one of the main prerequisites being an ideal labial shoulder preparation. A 90-degree angle with no bevel is preferred; an angle other than this could prevent obtaining a perfect seal.

Of the three methods for obtaining porcelain labial or buccal margins, the platinum foil matrix technique is perhaps the most accurate, producing perfectly sealed margins routinely. The next best method is the one that uses a high-fusing porcelain compound, and the least desirable method is the body porcelain-to-die technique.

Contour

Proper contour is a prime factor in a successful restoration. The dentist must communicate needed information to the laboratory technician in order to ensure a finished restoration that is both functionally and esthetically acceptable. This can be accomplished by communicating certain tangible guidelines that can be followed throughout the entire fabrication of the restoration.

"Every-Other-Tooth" Model

Once the dentist and patient have agreed upon a satisfactory provisional restoration, any one or several of the six anterior teeth can be used as a guide for the technician to follow during the fabrication of the final restoration. It shows the labial and incisal limits and can be used throughout the entire laboratory procedure, from waxing to full contour, to final porcelain contouring before glazing.

The every-other-tooth model can be derived from several sources: (1) prepared every-other-tooth model, (2) diagnostic model cutout, (3) provisional model cutout, and (4) waxed tooth with index.

Prepared "Every-Other-Tooth" Model (Fig 1-12)

An impression is made after preparing every other tooth. The model, with removable dies, is made from this impression and is used as a guide for waxing and contouring crowns individually. This method is used for cases where the restoration is patterned after the natural dentition where very little or no contour changes are necessary. This method is recommended when the patient and dentist are satisfied with the contour of the natural preoperative dentition, thus the dentist instructs the technician to duplicate tooth contour that was present before preparation.

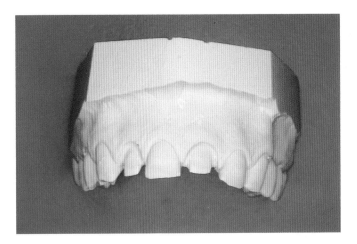

Fig 1-12 "Every-other-tooth" model. When preparing the teeth for this model, the dentist must decide which teeth will be of most help to the technician. As many of these as possible should be left intact, as long as they do not fall in the every-other-tooth preparation plan. For example, if six maxillary anterior teeth are to be restored, the dentist should select the least desirable teeth to prepare; however, they must fall in an every-other-tooth pattern.

Diagnostic Model Cutout

Closely related to the prepared every-other-tooth model is the diagnostic model of the unprepared teeth with a cutout tooth and index that can be used as a guide to duplicate the original contour. This is accomplished by cutting one tooth or several from the diagnostic model and attaching them to an index that can be transferred from the diagnostic cast to the master working model. The index must be made to fit unprepared posterior teeth that are not included in the treatment plan.

Provisional Model Cutout (Figs 1-13a to d)

If the diagnostic model is unacceptable for contour duplication, the provisional model may be considered in that contour improvements can be made not only before the provisional restoration but also after seating. Broken-down and missing teeth can be reconstructed and contoured on the diagnostic model to meet functional and cosmetic requirements. This model is used for constructing the provisional restoration, which is then further refined in the mouth. Only after the dentist and patient are satisfied should an impression be taken and attached to an index and used in the same manner as the diagnostic cutout model for contour duplication.

Waxed Tooth With Index

This method is appropriate when missing teeth are involved. The missing tooth is waxed and attached to an index that is interchangeable with the every-other-tooth and master working models. The tooth is waxed in the pontic area and is used as a guide for waxing the abutments. Missing teeth often initiate tooth movement, bringing about abnormally small or large spaces. This method gives the laboratory an opportunity to plan the width of not only the pontic but also the abutment teeth. In most cases such as this, compromises must be made as to size and contour to fill these spaces while satisfying esthetic demands.

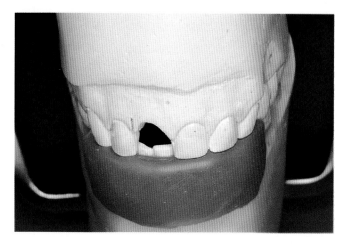

Fig 1-13a Mounted maxillary provisional model with right central incisor cut out. When cutting a tooth from a provisional model, take care not to interfere with the gingival tissue. The stone tooth can be mounted to an index, or a tooth can be waxed in its place and mounted. If slight contour improvements are desired, a waxed version may be more appropriate. (Note anterior index used to provide exact incisal edge position and contour for eventual waxed tooth.)

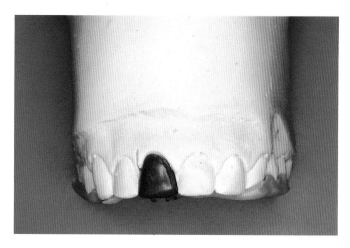

Fig 1-13b Waxed maxillary right central incisor on cutout of provisional model. The tooth is waxed to the anterior index and contoured to meet functional and esthetic needs. Then it is attached to a hard wax index that is seated securely onto unprepared posterior teeth. (Prepared posterior teeth can also be used for this purpose if they are included in the treatment plan but can be used only before posterior restorations are seated.)

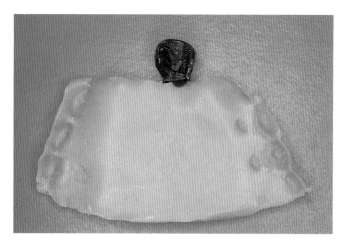

Fig 1-13c Waxed central incisor attached to index. Note definite posterior seat that fits onto the occlusal surface of the posterior teeth. The index with the waxed tooth is used throughout the entire fabrication of the restoration. It works best for cases that involve individual anterior restorations but can be used to some extent for a multiple-unit restoration in which the units are cast in one solid substructure.

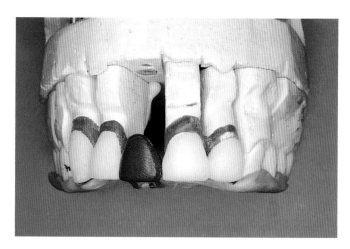

Fig 1-13d Waxed maxillary right central incisor with index during final contouring of five anterior teeth. This waxup helps greatly for restoring labial contour of the provisional restoration. The *left central incisor* is contoured to complement the waxed right central incisor restoration and the *left lateral incisor*.

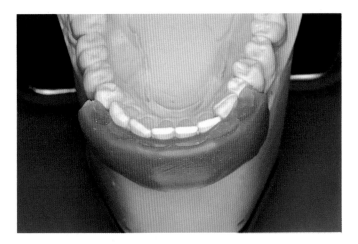

Fig 1-14a A wax anterior incisal index derived from occluding the model of the provisional restoration. Although a silicone or rubber-base material is usually preferred, occasionally the flexibility of these materials create problems and a more stable material is better suited (ie, hard wax or stone). Regardless of which material is used, a sharp, clear impression of the incisal edges of the maxillary anterior teeth should be obtained, making sure that the maxillary and mandibular models are properly occluded.

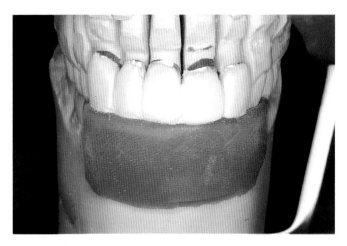

Fig 1-14b Completed prefired porcelain buildup with anterior incisal index. The index was used throughout the entire laboratory procedure, that is, waxing to full contour, metal substructure evaluation after casting, and during the application of four layers of porcelain (opaque, transition layer, body, and enamel). The index shows available space at the conclusion of each stage. (Note platinum foil at shoulder area used to obtain porcelain labial margins.)

Anterior Incisal Index (Figs 1-14a to e)

The incisal edge of the anterior restoration is the most critical in regard to function, esthetics, and patient comfort. Its position and contour play an integral role in phonetics in that the tongue and lips must be allowed to maneuver freely and combine their efforts to ensure authentic sounds. When the incisal edge of the restoration is altered in length or position from either the diagnostic or corrected provisional model, ideal phonetics may be hindered.

The lower lip is exceptionally sensitive to the feel of the incisal edge of the maxillary anterior teeth. Any change in length or position is readily detected, and often the patient will register a complaint.

Incisal length and position of both the maxillary and mandibular anterior teeth are also important

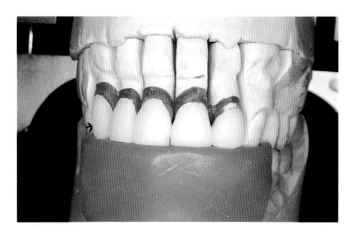

Fig 1-14c Contoured anterior restorations, using the anterior incisal matrix to verify crown length. The matrix and anterior guide table (when articulator is in protrusive position) will act as a reference for proper crown length. With reasonable care during fabrication, the anterior incisal matrix and guide table should coincide. If they don't, steps should be taken to correct the discrepancy.

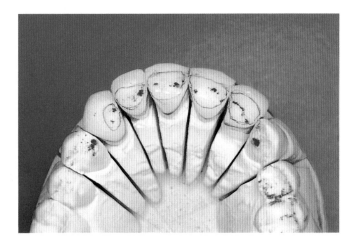

Fig 1-14d Lingual view of preglazed restorations. The lingual incisal edges were formed by the anterior incisal index while the anterior guide table dictated the remaining lingual surfaces. Note definite centric stops that are essential for preventing the teeth from extruding. This is especially important when individual units are involved. Connected units create less problems while keeping the teeth immobile. (When lingual areas are too thin to accommodate porcelain coverage, metal stops should be considered.)

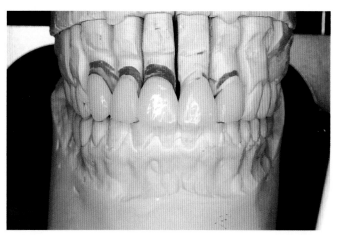

Fig 1-14e Five maxillary anterior restorations, glazed and ready for seating. Using the anterior incisal index the dentist and technician can verify that the crown length, incisal edge position, and contour are correct because the index is an exact registration of that found on the provisional restoration. Further, it ensures optimum phonetics, function, and esthetics.

for incising food. Any deviation associated with either could interrupt this and indirectly be the cause of future ailments.

Most problems having to do with length and position associated with the maxillary and mandibular anterior teeth can be prevented or resolved by incorporating an anterior incisal index into the treatment plan. It can be constructed with any material that is capable of registering the incisal edges of anterior teeth. Although wax or stone is acceptable, any of the silicone-type impression materials are preferred.

The index is taken from the corrected mounted diagnostic or provisional model. The dentist must decide the best source for the index. The diagnostic model may require the filling of the pontic areas and occlusal adjustments prior to constructing the index. The provisional restoration is a more appropriate source in that upon seating, further functional and esthetic refinements can be

made before a model is poured. The dentist may elect to have the patient wear the provisional restoration for several weeks, making changes and refinements until both are absolutely satisfied that optimum function and esthetics have been attained before the index is formed. Only then should an impression be made and a model poured of the provisional restoration.

The model is mounted on the articulator, using the same method for articulating and maintaining the vertical dimension and any other measurement used for mounting the master working model. The material is mixed to a putty consistency and applied to the maxillary and mandibular anterior teeth. If the maxillary anterior teeth are to be involved in the restoration, their labial surfaces are exposed, leaving just the incisal edges in the compound. If the mandibular teeth are to be restored, only the incisal edges are duplicated in the impression.

When properly prepared, the anterior incisal index dictates the exact length and incisal edge position of the anterior teeth that will be included in the restoration. The index is used first in waxing to full contour, establishing the correct labial and incisal aspect. The lingual functional contour is developed in conjunction with the anterior guide table. When the wax is fully contoured, the available thickness for metal substructure and porcelain, both labially and lingually, should be checked. If insufficient thickness is available for metal and porcelain lingually, metal stops should be considered. It is important at this time to decide whether it is practical to use porcelain in this area. Otherwise, the restoration could be completed with a porcelain lingual surface that is too thin to withstand normal function, eventually resulting in fracture or wear into the opaque, either of which is undesirable. Only when sufficient thickness is available (0.5 mm minimum, excluding metal thickness) should porcelain be selected for the lingual surface. Metal thickness in this area will depend on the type of alloy used.

The labial, incisal, and interproximal surfaces of the restoration are cut back until enough wax is uniformly removed to allow for an even thickness of porcelain (1 mm). The anterior incisal index is used as a reference to ensure accurate measurement. It is also used when applying porcelain, allowing the ceramist to gauge layer thickness after each application. This is especially helpful in establishing enamel thickness and designating precise areas for specific irregularities. Without this guide, the restoration could be overbuilt, requiring extra grinding that could result in the removal of needed color and characterization. Before glazing the restoration, the index is used to ensure proper length and incisal edge position. It gives the ceramist an opportunity to make necessary changes before final glaze.

If the dentist does not supply an anterior incisal index, the laboratory technician should request one or should fabricate one in the laboratory, using the above information in order to ensure accurate results. Without such a guide it is impos-

sible for a technician to know tooth length and incisal edge position.

Tissue Model (Figs 1-15a to m)

Because the dies and model are trimmed such that papillae and gingivae are eliminated, it is impossible for the technician to properly contour a restoration on the trimmed master working model that will conform with tissue location. To compensate for this tissue loss, a model is fabricated with the sole purpose of showing tissue arrangement, thus its name: *tissue model*. The tissue model, like the every-other-tooth model and anterior incisal index, should be used throughout the entire fabrication of the restoration. The case is waxed to full contour on the master working model and transferred to the tissue model; this will assure the technician it is not over- or undercontoured. Overcontouring will cause impingement in the mouth, resulting in eventual tissue damage. Undercontouring will leave unsightly spaces that most patients object to. Food traps and phonetic difficulties could also occur in an undercontoured restoration.

By following the tissue model, the boundaries of the restoration will fall within the limits of the tissue, deriving not only an esthetic advantage but also contributing to its health.

The tissue model can be fabricated in several ways, using materials most convenient to the dentist and laboratory staff. A stone model can be duplicated from the master working model before the dies are cut and trimmed. The dies are pinned so that each can be cut and removed. This is an advantage in that each unit can be contoured individually. The disadvantage, however, is that the tissue area is inflexible.

Another method involves constructing a stone model with a flexible material in the tissue area. The flexible material is placed into an alginate impression in just the areas associated with the restoration. Retention loops are embedded and the balance is poured in stone. The advantage with

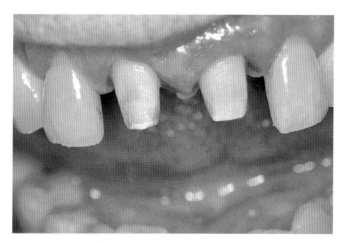

Fig 1-15a Prepared maxillary central incisors, ready for impressions. Usually, extreme care is taken in producing ideal preparations with flawless impressions and precise working dies and models, but all too often tissue location and contour are overlooked. Tissue health and maintenance are just as important as a functionally and esthetically sound restoration. In order to satisfy this need, the dentist must supply the technician with the information that will be incorporated into the fabrication of the restoration and ensure healthy gingival tissue.

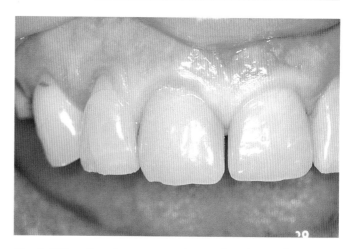

Fig 1-15b Poorly contoured completed maxillary central incisor restorations that cannot be seated because of tissue interference. Note tissue impingement, which, if overlooked, could cause eventual damage in this area. Although these restorations are functionally and esthetically sound, they are unacceptable and must be refabricated. A model showing tissue location would have helped prevent this from occurring. A tissue model should accompany every case, whether constructed in the dental office or in the laboratory.

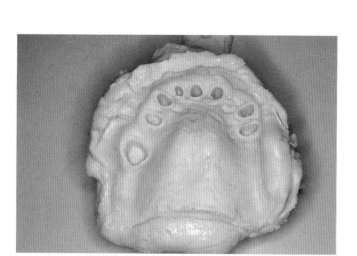

Fig 1-15c Alginate impression of master model before the dies were trimmed and with gingival tissue still intact. When using a flexible material (silicone or rubber base) for the tissue model, alginate or hydrocolloid must be used. For a stone tissue model, all impression materials are adaptable. (Alginate and hydrocolloid impressions must be poured immediately.)

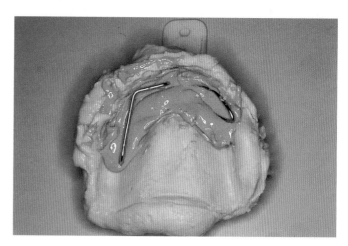

Fig 1-15d Silicone material with wire retention. The material is vibrated into the impression just in the area around the prepared teeth. Some flexible materials are more difficult to flow than others. These materials should be "teased" and vibrated to prevent trapped air that could cause bubbles. A wire retention (paper clip) is inserted (before the material matures) to act as a retention for the stone part of the model.

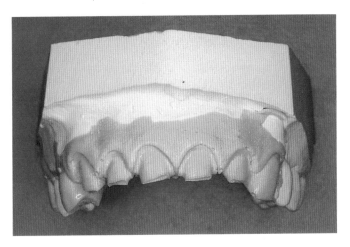

Fig 1-15e Completed tissue model. The second half of the model is poured in stone and trimmed. There are two minor disadvantages with this type model, however. First, the dies are somewhat flexible and may cause slight distortion in some cases. Second, the dies cannot be removed for individual consideration. When needed, there are alternatives for each (see Figs 1-15f and 1-15g).

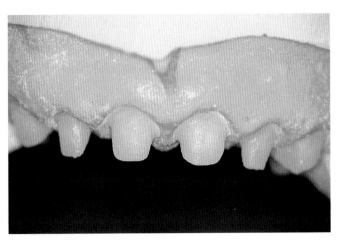

Fig 1-15f Tissue model with acrylic resin dies. If it is anticipated that the flexible die will be a problem, this type of model should be constructed. The working dies are poured in acrylic resin (multi-unit) with retention. Then, flexible material is poured into only the working tissue areas. Retention loops are embedded into the material to serve as connectors with the final stone sections. In this type of model, the dies will not flex and the restorations will have a more definite seat.

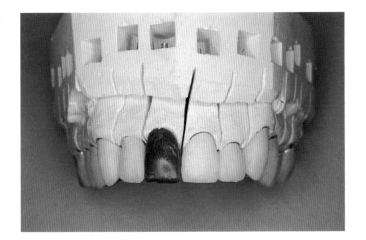

Fig 1-15g Stone tissue model. When special attention is required for each die, a stone tissue model is constructed so that each die is removable. The advantage of this type of model is that wax can be applied directly; with a flexible-type material, the wax pattern must be transferred from the master working model.

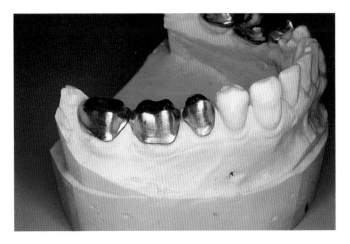

Fig 1-15h A solid stone tissue model with castings seated in place. The tissue model is important not only for the waxing and final contour, but also for the casting stage to verify margin fit and prevent over- or undercontouring in the tissue area. Both the buccal (labial) and lingual surfaces must be examined before applying porcelain. The model will indicate any necessary adjustment.

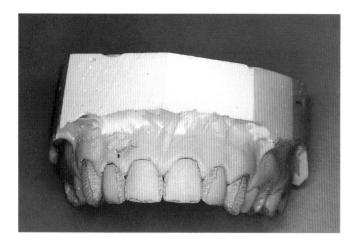

Fig 1-15i Maxillary tissue model with seated restorations being contoured before glaze. An undercontoured restoration is just as undesirable as one that is overcontoured at the gingival area. Undercontoured tissue areas of a restoration will leave unsightly spaces that could cause phonetic and esthetic problems. Most patients will complain, and with good reason. In some cases it is impossible to completely fill these spaces. Space size should be kept to a minimum, however. The tissue model will help determine this.

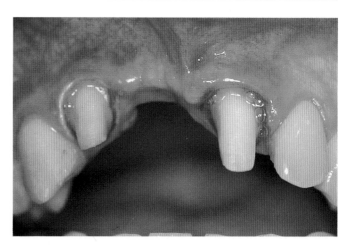

Fig 1-15j Prepared maxillary right lateral and left central incisors after extraction of right central incisor. When the three-unit bridge is eventually seated, the pontic area must be esthetically restored. An improperly contoured pontic could cause tissue damage and/or bring about unhygienic conditions by trapping food and making this area impossible to keep clean. A tissue model can help solve this potential problem.

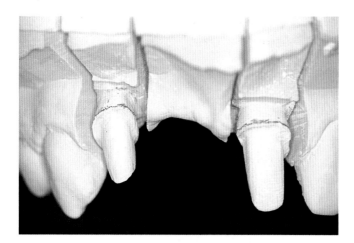

Fig 1-15k Pontic areas usually create problems during the fabrication of a restoration under normal circumstances and more so when much model trimming is required, as in this case. The technician has no way of knowing the exact tissue boundaries in this area; therefore, it is impossible to wax the pontic precisely without contour guidelines to follow.

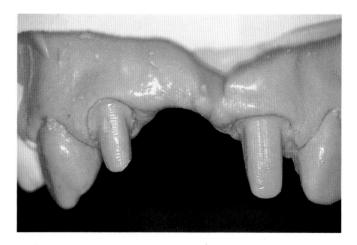

Fig 1-15l Tissue model (see also Figs 1-15j and 1-15k). Labial view showing exact tissue location in both the pontic and die areas. The completed wax pattern (full contour) can be transferred from the master working model to the tissue model for evaluation of function and esthetics.

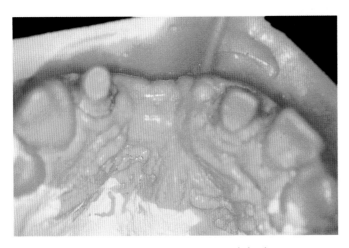

Fig 1-15m Lingual view of tissue model. There are several theories as to how the pontic should be contoured over the ridge. Lingually, most agree that it should be contoured to eliminate the possibility of tongue interference and/or trapping of food during mastication. While the lingual portion of the pontic may not be as important esthetically as the labial, a faulty contour in this area could cause the restoration to fail. It is necessary, therefore, that the technician know exact lingual tissue location.

this method is that the tissue area is flexible and greatly resembles mouth tissue in mobility and texture. The disadvantage is that this model cannot be separated into individual units but must be used as a solid model. Another disadvantage is that the dies are also flexible and could cause slight distortion when the restoration is seated. A third method, and probably the best of the three, involves dies poured in stone or acrylic resin, leaving the tissue portion free for the flexible

material. This model supplies rigid support for the restoration and flexibility in the tissue area, allowing for proper contour in wax, metal, and porcelain.

Solid Contact Model

A restoration, especially one involving several individual units, may fit the master working model perfectly, but when actually taken to the mouth, it may not fit. The dentist may then have to spend extra time adjusting contacts. The time lost could be costly and in most cases could be avoided if a solid contact model were used during the final stages of fabrication. Separated dies in the master working model permit slight movement, creating some question as to the exact tooth position in the mouth. A solid model, on the other hand, represents exact tooth location, thus permitting accurate contact adjustments in the laboratory. The solid model also represents a more accurate mesiodistal dimension of adjacent teeth not involved in the restoration.

When stone models are used, these teeth on the master working model will develop wear at the contact areas as the restored units are moved off and on. The wear on these teeth is significant enough to create a discrepancy between the working model and the mouth, thus requiring extra effort at the chair during seating. In almost every case, when transferring a restoration from the master working model to the solid model, some contact adjustment must be made before perfect seating can be accomplished.

The stone tissue model could be used as a solid contact model as well as a solid model duplicated from the master working model before the dies are cut and trimmed (Fig 1-16).

Color

Of all the information that must be communicated to the laboratory technicians, color is probably the most difficult. This is due primarily to the inadequacies of commercial shade guides. Much of the problem can be solved by using a more logical approach. The Four Dimensional Tooth Color System uses a customized tooth color guide to detect and measure the four tooth color dimensions (see Chapter 3).

Patient's Comments

Although "patient's comments" are last in order of importance in case planning, it should not be taken lightly; often a restoration is unacceptable to the patient simply because his or her requests during planning were ignored. Of course, it is not always possible to fully comply with all the requests made by the patient, but whenever possible, and if the requests fall within the treatment plan with no compromise to functional needs, the dentist should attempt to incorporate them. The dentist should carefully study the requests and relay the acceptable ones to the laboratory.

Some typical patient comments are: "I have gone for so many years with unsightly teeth, I want my new ones to be beautiful, white, and straight." "My teeth were very light when I was young; I want my 'caps' to look exactly like these pictures." A periodontally involved patient with no interproximal pappillae might say, "I want no spaces between my teeth." Requests such as these are unreasonable, of course, and to comply completely, with no regard to the patient's age and

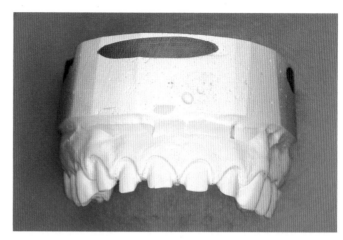

Fig 1-16 Solid contact model. A solid model of prepared teeth shows the technician exact tooth contact found in the mouth. It should be used as a final step before case delivery so that contact areas are not over- or under-contoured. The master working model is unreliable for this purpose because of die wear and movement. The solid stone contact model can also serve as a tissue model.

other circumstances, could mean fabricating an artifical-looking restoration that looks out of place. Many requests are not as unreasonable as the above, however, and in some cases can help the dentist decide on the best treatment plan.

It is important for the dentist to point out to the patient that the main concern is to restore the mouth to its fullest functional capacity and incorporate into the restoration as many requests as possible. The patient should be told that the most esthetic restorations are those that look most natural, and that the requirements for a natural-looking restoration will vary from patient to patient and be dictated by the remaining natural teeth. The closer the technician can approach the contour and color of the patient's remaining teeth, the more esthetic will be the completed restoration.

After the functional requirements have been recognized, the patient's comments should be evaluated. Again, whenever possible, the dentist should include these desires in the treatment plan, stipulating to the laboratory what is expected. Often, the laboratory can fabricate a restoration that incorporates all the needed ingredients for ideal function, contour, and color, and by altering contour and color enough to satisfy the patient, still deliver an acceptable restoration. It is much more gratifying to the dentist and laboratory technician to have a patient happy with the restoration rather than reluctantly accepting it with the idea that after awhile, he or she will get accustomed to it.

During my 35 years as a dental technician, I have been fortunate to have the opportunity to see patients before and after restoration completion. During color selection, I include every comment made by the patient on the information sheet with the color selection and laboratory procedures prescribed for that patient. During planning and fabrication, if a decision must be made regarding color or contour, one of the patient's comments may help me. In my experience, whenever it is possible to comply even partially with the desires of the patient, the completed restoration will be more acceptable to the patient.

Unfortunately, most dental technicians today do not have the luxury of a close relationship with dentist and patient. Unless the technician is located in the dental office, communication must be carried out by phone or written correspondence. This does not mean that close communication should not be pursued. When it is not possible to have the technician present, the dentist should consult the laboratory by phone before promising the patient a given restoration if there is a doubt as to whether or not the laboratory can produce it. Once the laboratory staff assures the dentist it can fabricate the desired restoration, the dentist can begin collecting all the information that must be communicated to the laboratory, including the patient's comments.

Case planning, therefore, is the keystone to the entire treatment. It puts the dentist, laboratory, and patient in tune with each other and is essential to help ensure optimum results.

Conclusion

The quality of a dental restoration depends greatly on how well the dentist and technician communicate. Each is responsible for supplying the other with certain information and guidelines. The laboratory staff must have as much information as possible from the dentist. Much of this is in the form of models and written instruction. The dentist needs input from the laboratory as to feasible materials and techniques available for each restoration.

Chapter 2

Metal Substructure: Design and Alloy Selection

Very often, esthetic-conscious dentists and technicians will overlook the most critical component of a ceramic restoration: the metal substructure. It is a well-established fact that function is more important that contour and color in any given restoration. It is impossible to define function without including the metal substructure; its physical and chemical makeup and its design mark the beginning for the functional aspect of the restoration. To obtain optimum function, accurate alloy selection and substructure design must be made during case planning. Several factors, which vary with the needs of each case, will influence this decision. Careful evaluation should be made with input from the laboratory.

Factors that must be addressed while keeping in mind the projected acceptable esthetic result include: (1) needed hardness and strength for the restoration, (2) the effect the restoration will have on opposing dentition, and (3) general health of the patients' gingivae, periodontal tissue, and bone.

Substructure Design

When in doubt as to the occlusal and functional needs of a particular case, the restoration should be waxed to full contour (Fig 2-1a). After the fully waxed case has been adjusted and contoured to fulfill these requirements, it should be cut back to an ideal design (Fig 2-1b). Just enough wax should be removed to accommodate an even thickness of porcelain (1 mm); porcelain strength decreases with thickness greater than 1 mm. Care should be taken on individual units to supply sufficient interproximal metal support for porcelain (Figs 2-1c and d). There should be adequate metal thickness in areas where greater stresses are anticipated. For example, milled areas for removable partial dentures (Fig 2-1e) and connections for precision attachments (Fig 2-1f) should be bulky enough to withstand abnormal stress loads. Sufficient wax should be removed with proper design when porcelain margins are involved. Care must be taken in multiunit restorations to supply enough interproximal thickness for strength yet leave enough space to prevent gingival impingement (Fig 2-1g).

Alloy Systems

During the early days of porcelain-to-metal fabrication, not many alloy systems were available. The most widely used and the only system that produced acceptable results was the *precious alloy system*. Although the precious alloys met general requirements for an acceptable restoration, they lacked in other areas. Eventually it became evident that there was a need for other systems to support functional stresses that precious alloys were not capable of supplying. Even though precious alloys are still the most widely used, newer systems with many advantages have become popular in recent years.

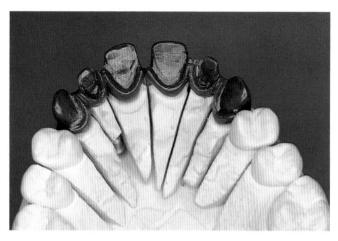

Fig 2-1a A well-designed metal substructure begins with a full waxup that shows what the restoration will eventually be. A uniform cutback of approximately 1 mm will supply the porcelain with a substructure that will promote maximum compression strength and ideal support throughout.

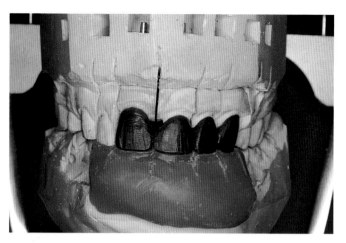

Fig 2-1b To ensure that individual units have interproximal support, each unit must be waxed to full contour, establishing functional and esthetic needs that include incisal edge position, labial contour, mesial and distal boundaries, and anterior guidance.

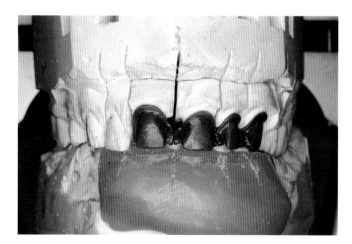

Fig 2-1c Once the waxing requirements have been fulfilled with the help of the incisal index and anterior guide table, each waxed unit is cut back uniformly, contouring interproximally so that maximum porcelain support will be incorporated into the metal substructure. The margins are then refined and the wax patterns sprued, invested, and cast.

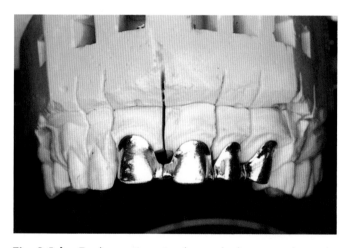

Fig 2-1d Each casting is dressed down and made ready to accept porcelain. During this procedure care must be taken to maintain the interproximal support that was waxed into each unit; overzealous grinding could quickly remove this. Once this, along with the other functional requirements, has been examined, the castings are ready for porcelain application.

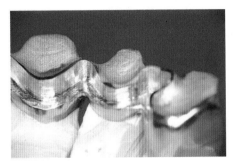

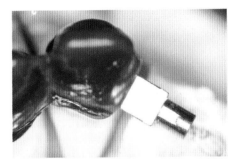

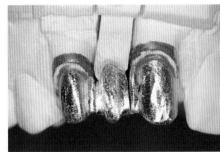

Fig 2-1e

Fig 2-1f

Fig 2-1g

Fig 2-1e Often, a restoration is made up of a combination of fixed and removable partial dentures. The fixed partial denture must be designed to support all the forces exerted upon it by the removable partial denture. One such restoration is the milled removable partial denture that depends on the milled walls of the fixed partial denture for retention and load distribution. The walls and interproximal areas must be bulky enough to withstand all forces directed to them, with no chance of distortion or fracture.

Fig 2-1f The walls of the restoration that will eventually support a precision attachment must be waxed bulky enough to absorb all forces directed there by the removable partial denture. Semiprecision and dovetail attachments should have the same consideration. If this is neglected during the waxing stage, the restoration is likely to fail.

Fig 2-1g Porcelain margins should be prepared for during the wax cutback so that the castings will need minimum grinding. This is especially true in restorations with precious alloy understructures; it could be quite costly in time and material. In multiunit restorations, whether cast together or postsoldered, care must be taken that the metal not impinge on gingival tissue.

In order for the dentist and technician to make the best possible choice when selecting an alloy for a particular metal substructure, they should know what each system has to offer and its advantages and disadvantages. Obviously, the system that can provide the most advantages should be used. The needs for each case are based on: interproximal connections; labial or buccal and lingual thicknesses; functional responsibilities; precision attachment and dovetail involvement; beveled margins; anterior lingual stops; opposing dentition; occlusal contour; and path of insertion. The compounds that make up the alloys are called upon to satisfy these needs.

High-Gold-Content Alloys (Noble Metal)

High-gold-content alloy (gold: 84%/platinum: 7.9%/palladium: 4.6%) was one of the earliest alloys to be developed and is probably the least complicated in that it has good castability properties and bonds well with porcelain. It is corrosion resistant, nontoxic, and soft enough for fine occlusal adjustment. Its yield strength and modulus of elasticity are acceptable for most restorations. Finishing and polishing are easy, producing a brilliant luster.

This alloy system does have disadvantages, however, the greatest being its relative softness.

This characteristic is responsible for its low sag resistance, which can be troublesome during porcelain fabrication. Under microscopic scrutiny, almost every restoration with high-gold content will show some degree of sag even though in most cases the discrepancy is acceptable.

Another problem associated with its softness is the difficulty in dressing down the metal for porcelain application; finishing stones will tend to roll the outer skin and trap contaminants rather that flake them off, as found in harder alloys. Many time this cannot be seen with or without the aid of a microscope. These contaminants will eventually surface during porcelain fabrication in the form of bubbling or porosity and could reach the point of porcelain fracture caused by the formation of gases that are brought about by the combustion of these contaminants.

Possibly the most frustrating situation arises after completing a beautiful, well-engineered restoration only to find part of the beveled margin polished away. This is due to the relative softness of the alloy and leaves no alternative other than to reconstruct the restoration. This is time-consuming and expensive for the laboratory staff and dentist. In spite of the several disadvantages this alloy system possesses, it is still the favorite of many dentists and technicians and will always be a viable choice when a relatively soft substructure is needed.

Low-Gold-Content Alloys

Formula changes were eventually made to high-gold-content alloys. The gold content was lowered from 84% to 50% while the silver content was raised from 1.3% to 12% and palladium was raised from 4.6% to 30%. This change in formula brought about several significant advantages over the high-gold-content alloy. The higher melting temperature (1,200°C to 1,260°C) lessened the possibility of metal sag and distortion during porcelain fabrication and increased the strength in longer spans. The low-gold-content alloy presented a better environment for dressing down the casting in that its increased hardness lent to grindings flaking off rather than rolling and trapping contaminants, thus preventing porcelain bubbling and fracturing. Its increased hardness also decreased the possibility of damage and wear to the delicate bevel at the margin. Low-gold-content alloy retained the nontoxic property of high-gold-content alloy. Further, its lower price established a welcomed relief from rising gold prices.

Some disadvantages were introduced; however, the increased silver content presented the possibility of "greening" the porcelain, and changes had to be made in the opaque procedure to overcome the grayness created by the increased amounts of palladium and silver. Opaque porcelain was originally formulated to block out the influence derived from high-gold-content alloys. The same opaque formula could not sufficiently compensate for the lack of gold color in the newer alloy.

The formulae of new low-gold-content alloys have since been changed to help solve the color problems found in older systems. Most porcelain manufacturers have changed opaque and body porcelain formulas to prevent "greening" and reduce grayness (lower value) when used with these alloys. These improvements on the part of both the alloy and porcelain manufacturers have made this alloy system more attractive to both the dentist and technician and thus an excellent alternative when high-gold-content alloy is not feasible for a particular restoration.

No-Gold-Content Alloys (Base Metal Alloys)

Soon after the advent of porcelain-to-metal, it became evident that the noble metal alloys could be improved in several areas. The increase in silver and palladium did indeed improve its performance as a substantial substructure, yet further improvements were made in the form of a *base metal alloy*. The most common base metal alloy used today is a nickel-chromium combination with a host of trace elements; the percentage of each varies with the alloy and is regulated by the manufacturer. The main difference between base metal alloys is the presence or absence of beryllium. Some believe that in spite of its usefulness, beryllium should be eliminated from the alloy because of its potential health hazards to laboratory technicians. Others feel its presence in the alloy is essential. Beryllium contributes to flowability during casting and aids in oxidation control. Beryllium plays an integral role in base metal alloys, and to eliminate it from the formula would compromise the alloy's efficiency.

No gold-content alloys (base metal alloys) are very useful in those cases where high- and low-gold-content alloys lack necessary strength and hardness. A base metal alloy should be considered for restorations that could otherwise fail due to a substructure not able to withstand excessive forces and wear. However, base metal alloys, like high-gold-content alloys, do have some disadvantages that should be recognized. Compare the two alloy systems before making a selection for any given restoration.

High-Gold-Content Alloy (Noble Metal) vs No-Gold-Content Alloy (Base Metal Alloy)

Noble metal and base metal alloys represent two alloy types with extremely different physical and chemical characteristics. When selecting an alloy, characteristics of each should be considered. They include ease of controlling quality, the need for hardness and strength, the effect each has on surrounding tissue and wear to opposing dentition, veneer thickness advantage, pre- and post-fabrication connections, economy, and the effect the presence of nickel has on the patient and the potential health hazard beryllium has on the technician.

Quality Control

In order for any material or procedure to reach its optimum potential, quality control is imperative. Each material used in the fabrication of the restoration must be analyzed and properly used so that the end result is predictable.

Quality control begins in the operatory with tooth preparation and must be carried through until the completed restoration is seated. Some areas are more critical than others depending on the alloy used. The accuracy of fit in any restoration, regardless which alloy is used, depends solely on quality control exercised in the operatory through to the pouring of the dies. From the poured dies to the completed restoration, quality control takes on a different significance that does depend greatly on the alloy used for the substructure.

Quality control is more critical for base metal than for noble metal alloys. During the early and mid 1950s, when porcelain-to-metal fabrication began, quality was difficult to control, mainly because of the newer and unfamiliar materials required for this. Spruing, investing, and casting techniques had to be augmented to accommodate these new materials so that they could produce the most accurate restoration possible. Formulas and ingredients were changed to help eliminate problems as they occurred. In the case of noble metal alloys, it can be safely stated that all of the problems and inadequacies have been overcome. Quality control is now routine and results are fully predictable.

On the other hand, because there is a wide variety of base metal alloys on the market today, with varying ingredients, special attention is required in almost every phase of base metal alloy fabrication. For example, sprues must be precisely located to promote more efficient metal flow during casting because base metal alloys are sluggish. Investments must be able to accommodate higher burnout temperatures, and longer burnout time is required than that used for noble metal alloy. Care must be taken to not interfere

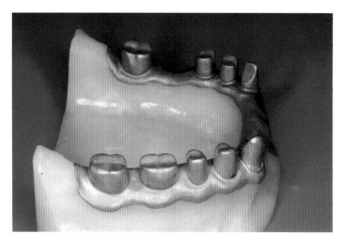

Fig 2-2a A solid cast model (with immovable dies) could be used to maintain quality control when evaluating an alloy. This is especially helpful when attempting to establish guidelines for processing a particular base metal alloy before using it for a metal substructure in an actual restoration. Cast metal dies (chrome-cobalt) are wear resistant and will remain accurate almost indefinitely.

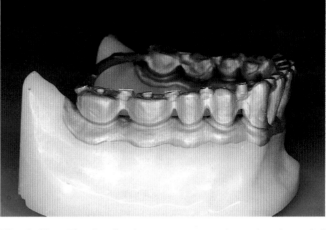

Fig 2-2b The finished casting is transferred to the solid evaluation model after the sprues and vents have been cut away and cleaned with 25-μm aluminum oxide spray. The casting must be completely free of investment that could prevent seating. Care must be taken to retain all finely beveled margins during this procedure so that if a flawed or incomplete margin is discovered after seating it can be credited to a faulty casting technique. The casting must not be forced onto the model; only slight finger pressure should be necessary for seating.

with the elements placed in the alloy to promote proper flowability and oxidation required for maximum porcelain bonding. Casting procedures are critical because of flowability and melting temperature. Further, melting temperature is difficult to determine, and if not accurately controlled, overheating could occur, resulting in elements being depleted thus creating an imbalance in the alloy.

Mismanagement of any procedure described above could result in an unacceptable restoration; ie, poor fit, undefined margins with lack of sharpness, porosity, and improper oxidation needed for adequate bonding with porcelain could result. Yet despite the shortcomings of base metal alloys, great strides made in research and development in recent years have made them a feasible material for supporting porcelain. Quality can be maintained routinely simply by paying careful attention to each phase. Before a labora-

tory attempts to make available a base metal system to its dentists, it should take steps to improve and stabilize quality control for each alloy it intends to use. Some sort of solid case or silver-plated model should be used for measuring the accuracy of trial castings. The solid model represents the mouth, eliminating chance of error that could be brought about by movement of individual dies (Figs 2-2a to g). Cast or silver-plated dies are used to prevent any possible dimensional change due to abrasion. The solid model should be constructed with utmost accuracy because acceptance of the quality controlled casting will depend on how well it adapts to this model. If the model is inaccurate, the evaluation will have been in vain.

Manufacturers' directions should be followed concerning waxing, spruing, investing, burnout, and casting. If, when transferring the finished casting from the master working model to the

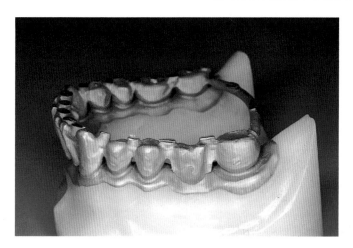

Fig 2-2c   If each stage of fabrication was properly carried out, the casting should seat well with no distortion or casting flaws. Close examination for any gross imperfections should be made. If the casting is satisfactory based on normal visual scrutiny, it should be examined further under a microscope; each unit should be checked separately for marginal fit and possible flaws. Should each unit of the casting pass the microscope examination, the procedures can be considered successful, assuring the technician that the entire method, from waxing to casting, can be used routinely with confidence.

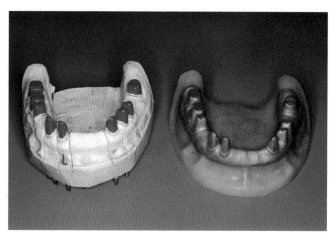

Fig 2-2d   The solid model is an exact duplicate of the master working model without die separation. The master model is prepared and treated in the same manner as performed for an actual case; dies are cut and separated, margins are trimmed under a microscope, and four thin layers of liquid spacer are applied to each die. When die spacer is completely dry, lubricant is applied and waxing begins.

Fig 2-2e   If after several trial castings, misfitting castings persist, a new casting should be made and placed onto the solid model before the sprues and vents are removed. The casting can then be evaluated with sprues and vents in place and a determination can be made as to whether or not the spruing and/or venting system is at fault. If, for example, the anterior section of the casting fits well but the posterior section is not seating properly, the problem can usually be directed to the spruing system. With the sprues in place, it gives the technician an opportunity to follow the metal flow and redesign the spruing system to overcome the problem in future castings.

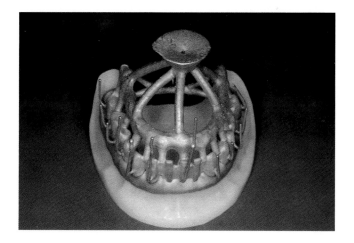

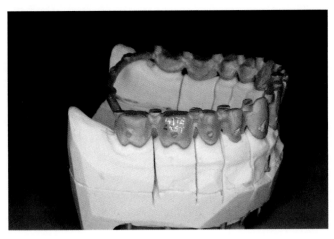

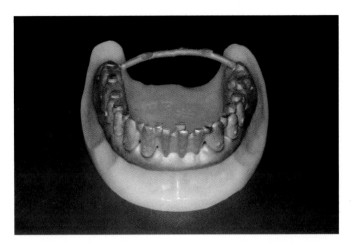

Fig 2-2f Should the casting seat satisfactorily on the master working model but not on the solid model, chances are good that a die could have shifted or become deformed. This denotes that the problem is probably not due to a faulty casting system but rather to negligence during die preparation and waxing. If this was an actual case, therefore, even though it fit the master working model well, it would not seat properly in the mouth and would be unacceptable. Note the bar connecting to two molars; if the metal substructure is not to be tried in the mouth, it remains on the casting until the restoration is completed. It helps prevent distortion during porcelain firing and gives the ceramist a convenient handle during porcelain application.

Fig 2-2g If the casting seats as well on the solid model as it does on the master working model, chances are good that both the waxing and casting systems used for that specific alloy are accurate and can be used reliably for an actual restoration. However, spruing, investing, and casting procedures may vary with different alloys; techniques proven successful for one alloy may not produce the same results for another.

solid quality control model the results are unsatisfactory, steps should be taken to eliminate the cause. These results should be examined under a microscope; what may appear to be acceptable with the naked eye may indeed be unacceptable after viewing under a microscope.

Because quality is more difficult to control when dealing with base metal alloys than with noble metal alloys, extra effort must be made to derive the same accuracy found with noble metal alloys. When this is accomplished, the results are gratifying. If problems occur, however, one must search for the cause of these problems.

Searching for the Cause of Casting Failures

Perhaps the greatest aid in searching for the cause of failure in a casting is the microscope (Fig 2-3). The search should begin with a thorough examination of the inner surface of the casting for nodules or deformities that could prevent the casting from seating completely. If the microscope reveals this, each nodule should be carefully removed, taking care not to damage the margins. This initial step should be taken for every casting before attempting to seat it on either the master working or solid model. After the interfering nodules are

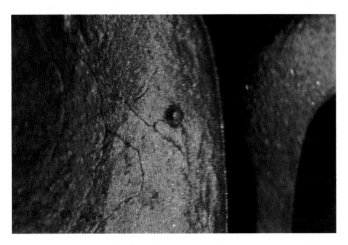

Fig 2-3 A search for the cause of a casting problem should begin with a microscope. A small nodule or slight deformity on the inner surface of the casting could prevent it from seating completely onto the master working model. Often the nodule is so small it is unrecognizable and very difficult to locate until examination is made with a microscope. A microscope is an essential piece of equipment and should be found in every laboratory; without its assistance, many problems could go unsolved.

removed, the casting should be tried on the master working model and once again examined under the microscope. Individual castings are uncomplicated to examine because problems are localized. A multiunit casting, however, is more complex and the cause could originate from several different areas. For example, warpage and distortion, which can take place in several locations on a multiunit casting due to ultrathin or thick walls, could be difficult to locate and troublesome to correct. Large pontic areas that span several tooth widths, bulky connections and lingual surfaces, thin labial or buccal surfaces, and heavy cusp tips are other examples of potential trouble spots that could create problems in seating.

Even when you follow the manufacturer's directions for handling investments and alloys, occasionally the results are unacceptable. Each procedure must be analyzed, revising each step until satisfactory results are obtained. Assuming that the dies and model are accurate, the five procedures that must be further evaluated are (1) waxing, (2) spruing, (3) investing, (4) burnout, and (5) casting and will be discussed as follows.

Prewaxing Procedures

Obviously, a flawless casting begins with proper tooth preparations and impressions. The dentist must decide which type of tooth preparation will be appropriate for any given case and which impression technique will produce the most accurate results. Even though techniques and materials will vary, the main concern is to eventually create a die that is an exact duplicate of a prepared tooth. Equally important is a die system that uses materials (stone or plated) that will withstand fracture, wear, or distortion during case construction.

Occasionally it is impossible to obtain a preparation free from undercuts because of tooth position or breakdown. If the dentist does not compensate for these undercuts before taking the impression, the undercut in the die must be blocked out before waxing; wax patterns that are pulled over an undercut, regardless how minor, will distort and not regain their original form. A proper blockout material should be used; it should satisfy all aspects of waxing. It should not distort during waxing and should not react unfavorably with die spacer and separating medium.

It is a common practice to coat the die with a spacer. There are several types available and they all serve the same purpose; they supply space for cement, thus reducing the hydraulic pressure developed during seating of the restoration. It also provides slight leeway during seating that could prevent porcelain fracture (Figs 2-4a to c).

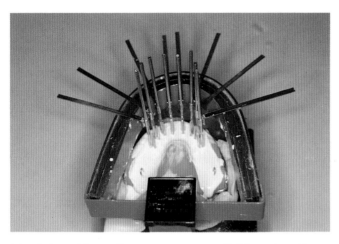

Fig 2-4a Many die systems are available today. Use a system that will best suit your needs while producing high-quality models and dies. It is impossible to fabricate an acceptable restoration on an inferior master working model with weak, loose dies. Multiunit restorations are especially affected; just a slight movement by any of the dies in the master working model could prevent the restoration from properly seating in the mouth.

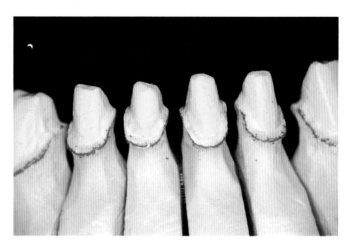

Fig 2-4b The dies in the master working model must be exact duplicates of the prepared teeth. The slightest distortion incorporated into any one of the dies will render the restoration unseatable, requiring a new impression and models. Dies should be handled carefully, keeping them free from abrasion and fracture.

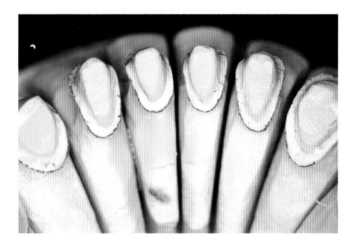

Fig 2-4c Each die should be inspected under a microscope and checked for flaws and undercuts. Flaws should be corrected and undercuts blocked out; afterwards, several applications of die spacer are made. The dies are now lubricated and made ready for waxing. In many laboratories the responsibility for fabricating dies and master working models is given to the employee with the least experience in dentistry. Often this person has recently been hired and knows little or nothing of the dental profession, much less the importance of accurate dies and master working models. Personnel in the die and model department of the laboratory should have special training; their work should be highly scrutinized and they should understand the importance of accuracy.

Waxing

Wax selection and manipulation should be the first area to be scrutinized when a casting fails. Waxes have been improved over the years and most in use today are of excellent quality. They must pass stringent tests to be accepted as a viable dental material. Problems, therefore, do not lie in its composition but in its manipulation. One of the greatest violations associated with wax manipulation is the tendency to not replace old wax with new. Adding new wax to the melting container will help maintain most of the required qualities, but completely replacing the old with new should be done routinely. This will ensure a more consistent quality control in the wax.

Proper manipulation is important in maintaining the integrity of the wax. When using the spatula technique, the wax should be heated uniformly and smoothly applied to a spacered, well-lubricated die, making sure not to incorporate folds into the wax pattern. When adding wax to a cooled pattern, care must be taken to heat the addition and the pattern uniformly to ensure a homogeneous union. The hot spatula should melt the pattern sufficiently so that the newly melted addition will flow into and combine with the pattern before cooling uniformly. This will help prevent inclusion of stresses and prevent flaking and voids, which could cause distortion and weakness. Stresses that are incorporated into the wax pattern will invariably be released in the form of distortion upon removing the pattern from the die. Even though the distortion may be slight, it could be enough to cause the casting to be unacceptable. In the case of multiunit casting, just one unit exhibiting this condition could prevent the entire casting from seating, thus leading to failure and loss of time and labor.

While it is important to heat the wax sufficiently for a homogeneous mix, overheating, whether it be in the spatula or in the melting unit, will alter the basic formula. This could burn off ingredients that are necessary to keep the wax free from distortion. Waxes kept at a temperature greater than that prescribed by the manufacturer over a long period of time will tend to separate and break down. This could cause certain ingredients to become volatile and others to settle to the bottom of the heating unit. A pattern made in this condition is subject to weakness and distortion and could result in an ill-fitting casting. Wax should be kept at the temperature prescribed by the manufacturer and never overheated.

Impurities. A factor often overlooked as a potential cause of casting failures is the inclusion of foreign materials in the wax. Airborne materials such as stone, metal, and porcelain grindings and any other dust particles found in the laboratory can easily find their way into the waxing unit if care is not taken to prohibit this. It is difficult to keep the melted wax covered during the waxing procedure and even more difficult to recognize these impurities. When they are included in the wax pattern, they may not be flushed away during burnout and could actually be incorporated into the casting. Depending on the impurities and the amount per given volume of alloy, the resulting effect could be serious. If enough impurities are incorporated into the alloy, it could cause a chemical imbalance that might alter the coefficient of expansion and eventually cause the porcelain to fracture. It could also cause the metal substructure to become brittle and weak, resulting in metal fracture at delicate connections. Further, it could create porous metal that might force gases into the porcelain during fabrication and interfere with the oxidation process necessary for optimum bonding of porcelain to metal.

It is essential, therefore, that wax be kept free from all foreign materials. This is difficult to maintain even in the cleanest laboratory. For this reason, it is important to periodically replace the old wax with new, taking care to keep it as free as possible from foreign material (Fig 2-5).

Surface texture. The finished wax pattern should be smooth and free of sharp corners. Any roughness on the surface of the wax or sharpness

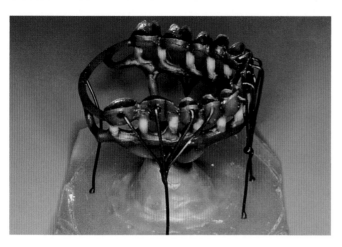

Fig 2-5 When a faulty substructure can be attributed to the waxing stage, several areas must be considered. The problem could occur anytime from the first wax application to the die to the spruing stage. Precautions should include fresh wax, uniform melting temperature, smooth, homogeneous application, and procedures to ensure it is contamination free. Improper wax manipulation will surely result in failure, because any discrepancy incorporated into the wax pattern before investing will be duplicated during casting.

around the edges could cause small pieces of investment to break off during casting due to the fast moving metal. Even though present day investments are much improved and more durable than the older types, there is always a possibility that tiny particles can be dislodged. When this happens, these particles can be trapped in the metal casting or be forced to the margin area. If particles of investment are trapped within the casting, they will invariably cause gassing during porcelain fabrication. Many times these particles are so small they can go unnoticed even in very thin veneer areas, but they will create damaging bubbling in the porcelain. Occasionally, degassing will expel some of the gases, but many times the gases will linger throughout the entire fabrication, periodically surfacing through the opaque and causing large bubblelike concavities that could be large enough to blow off the entire

porcelain veneer. When this occurs, many times the break through the opaque is so small it is almost unnoticeable, yet the force is almost enough to form a cavity several millimeters in diameter. This should be examined under a microscope and completely eliminated before attempting to repair the damage. Otherwise, it will continue to give off gas during each firing.

If these particles escape entrapment, they are often forced toward delicate margins by the swiftly moving molten metal, where they embed themselves to form ragged edges and cause short margins. This usually means having to redo the casting.

The wax pattern should be wiped free of surface roughness to eliminate sharp angles. This can be done by very carefully going over the entire surface with a fine piece of silk, being careful of margins and thin areas. This will give the wax surface a sheen and permit the investment to flow smoothly over the entire surface, thus permitting the molten metal to flow freely with no danger of breaking off particles of investment.

All of the above waxing requirements for quality control are equally important for both noble and base metal alloys. The only difference between the waxing procedures for the two alloys is the minimum thickness required for strength. The minimum thickness for a noble metal understructure is 0.3 mm. Areas thinner than this are prone to warpage during porcelain fabrication and fracture at interproximal connections. Base metal understructures need only a 0.1 mm thickness for maximum strength with no fear of warpage or fracture. These measurements should be made during the waxing procedure so as to eliminate the need for excessive grinding after casting.

To maintain optimum quality control in both noble and base metal alloy castings, there are certain basic fundamentals that must be applied in all five procedures: waxing, spruing, investing, burnout, and casting. Of the five, the one most common to both is waxing; waxing fundamentals and requirements are the same for each. In the other four procedures, although the fundamentals are basically the same, certain parameters must be augmented to ensure successful results when using base metal alloy.

Waxing to full contour. After applying a very thin layer of separating medium, the waxing begins. Of the several different waxing techniques, the most accurate and advantageous to good quality control is to wax to full contour. Waxing the restoration to full contour permits the technician to work in conjunction with the every-other-tooth model, an anterior index, a tissue model, and an anterior guide table. These added aids give the technician the exact guidelines necessary for a predictable result and complete control over quality. The every-other-tooth model dictates the labial contour, including mesial and distal boundaries. The anterior index indicates precise incisal edge position and contour, while the tissue model shows exact tissue location. Above all, the anterior guide table must be recognized as the basic functional guide in that it is used to duplicate the maxillary anterior lingual contour. Any waxing technique other than waxing to full contour cannot take full advantage of these aids. Although this holds true regardless of the alloy used, its significance is amplified when used with base metal alloys. If indeed a base metal substructure is more critical, making porcelain more vulnerable to fracture, the full waxing technique permits the technician to cut back just enough wax, evenly over the entire restoration, to ensure a uniform thickness of porcelain. This will provide sufficient metal support in all areas while creating proper contour for maximum compression strength, which is necessary for a ceramic restoration.

Along with full contour waxing, microscopic examination should be used to ensure that the wax pattern is free from folds, flaws, and voids. This holds true especially in the case of base metal substructure; the veneer surface of the casting will be approximately 0.1 mm thick, and even the slightest void in a casting this thin will weaken the restoration tremendously, creating a potential metal fracture under functional stress. The hardness of base metals makes it imperative that the casting require only minimal grinding and dressing down. Also, because even the finest margin cannot be burnished, it is essential that the wax pattern be exact with perfectly contoured margins.

Spruing

Spruing is a critical procedure regardless of which alloy is used, but it is even more critical with base metal alloy. The purpose of the sprue is to form a hollow path or channel for the molten metal to flow through from the crucible to the mold cavity. Proper gauge, length, direction, position, and attachment are essential for routine success. After wax elimination, the channel must provide the best route for the molten metal to take with the least amount of turbulence yet with sufficient force to fill the mold cavity perfectly. Spruing must be designed to comply with "cold" and "hot" spots in the mold and ideal locations for reservoirs. They must be located and contoured so the molten metal can flow smoothly with no sharp turns, so as to fill the mold completely, including very fine margins. The surface of the sprue should be glassy smooth and free of roughness that could cause turbulence or investment breakdown that might cause particles to be incorporated into the casting. Also, smooth rounded connections are essential to prevent this (Fig 2-6).

The spruing procedure for base metal alloy is more critical than for noble metal alloy. Lower specific gravity and the necessity for higher temperatures during casting make it imperative that sprue placement, gauge, and length be engineered so as to prevent miscasts.

Spruing must be designed to place the wax pattern in the proper position. McLean (1979) describes the significance of the "thermal zone" that is created upon cast completion and is located approximately in the center of the casting ring. The investment in this area will remain hotter than the surrounding areas, and the molten metal located here will solidify last. If the pattern is

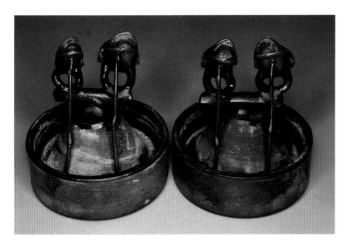

Fig 2-6 Finished wax patterns and sprues should be smooth and free of sharp edges. Molten metal should flow freely during casting. Unnecessary roughness could result in investment breakoff and entrapment. This could cause a porous substructure, incomplete and ragged margins, and a possible coefficient of expansion mismatch between the metal substructure and porcelain. These considerations should be made before investing, so as to ensure a smooth, accurate mold.

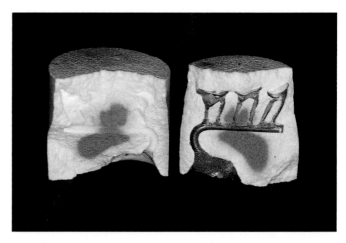

Fig 2-7 It is essential to place sprue and wax pattern in the casting ring to obtain a complete casting free of porosity. The "thermal zone" (the area of investment that cools last) plays a critical role during the casting procedure. The sprue or runner bar that supplies the casting with molten metal should be placed in the thermal zone while positioning the wax patterns on its periphery. The alloy, in this area, will remain molten long enough to supply needed flow to each unit, ensuring a complete, porous-free casting. If the wax patterns are placed in the thermal zone, the feeder bar may solidify before the casting, thus depriving it of alloy necessary for a complete casting.

placed directly in the center of the thermal zone, there is a great possibility that the feeder sprues will solidify before the casting, leaving the casting without a source of molten metal needed for completion. This would result in a porous casting, rounded margins, or a complete miscast, any of which is unacceptable. This theory holds true for both single-unit and multiple-unit castings.

Ideally, the sprues should be located as close to the center of the thermal zone as possible while locating the wax pattern on its periphery. This will permit the molten metal in the feeder sprues to remain molten longer, permitting them to feed the casting to completion. This ensures a porosity-free casting with sharp margins and less chance of a miscast. It not only produces a much stronger, better-fitting casting, but also one that will not interfere with porcelain fabrication. When multiple castings are involved, each wax pattern should be positioned equidistant from the center of the ring and in the same plane.

Even more important is positioning of bridges with pontics and heavy connections. If they are placed within the thermal zone, porous pontics and connections are almost sure to occur, causing weakness in the bridge and bubbling in the porcelain. Care should be taken, therefore, to place bulky areas away from the thermal zone, permitting feeder sprues to supply molten metal as needed to complete the casting (Fig 2-7).

Venting. With proper spruing for noble metal alloys, venting may not be necessary to remove lingering gases and heat that do not escape nor-

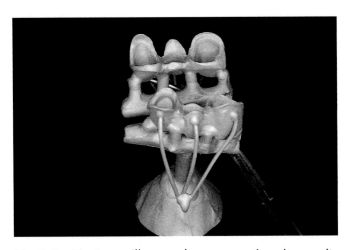

Fig 2-8 Venting will never harm a casting. It permits heat and gases to escape quickly and is beneficial in both heavy pontics and thin veneers. This is especially true in the case of base metal alloys where high heat and sluggish metal flow are prevalent. Venting could help prevent miscasts while promoting strong, dense, porous-free casting that will eventually help control porcelain quality. This is especially true when finely beveled margins are involved; venting ensures sharpness and accuracy.

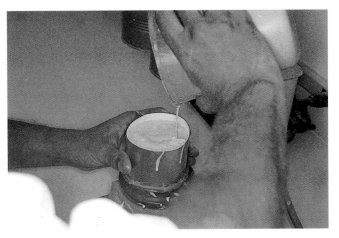

Fig 2-9 Investment techniques vary with materials and should coincide with the manufacturer's instructions. Prescribed powder-liquid ratio and spatulation time should especially be adopted. Even though the quality of investments has improved in recent years, close attention should be paid when selecting one for a particular alloy. Several investments may have to be tried before optimum results are achieved. Ill-fitting castings and fissures are a sign that the investment and/or investing technique should be evaluated. Base metal alloys are more technique sensitive than noble metal alloys and may require more attention in order to maintain good quality control.

mally through the investment. When in doubt, however, especially when fine-grain investments are used and the wax patterns are bulky, venting should be used.

When using base metal alloys, venting should be considered in cases where a dense casting is questionable (eg, where multiple units with bulky pontics are involved). A good rule to follow is: when in doubt, use vents. Venting cannot cause a case to fail but it could prevent a miscast and possible failure (Fig 2-8).

Investing

Investing procedures for noble and base metal alloys are essentially the same. The investments vary, however, and should be selected according to the alloy manufacturer's recommendations and used according to their specifications (Fig 2-9).

In the early years of porcelain-to-metal restorations when the only available substructure was noble metal alloy, investments were formulated to suit immediate needs. Some of the problems encountered were attributed to these investments (eg, ill-fitting castings, rough surface, dull and incomplete margins). Over the years, investment formulas have changed and noticeable improvement has made noble metal casting systems more controllable with greater predictability. Investments associated with base metal casting systems have been more of a problem because of the higher burnout and casting temperatures required. Improvements to these investments have been slower than with those used with noble metal alloys due to the large variety of base metal alloys on the market today. This adds to the difficulties in controlling quality in base metal alloy systems.

Wax Burnout

For both noble and base metal alloys, a two-stage wax burnout is recommended. A low first-stage temperature of approximately 500°F permits wax and plastic sprues to be eliminated more efficiently. This allows gases to escape more uniformly during casting. The first stage also eliminates water gradually in the form of steam, which could otherwise create tremendous internal pressure responsible for investment cracking and surface roughness. This is especially important when ringless casting systems are used. The first burnout stage should last approximately 15 minutes but should be extended when large bulky cases are involved (eg, a large ring with ten bulky wax patterns would need a longer first-stage burnout than a small ring with a few thin wax patterns). Wax burnout should never be rushed, especially in the first stage. Rapid first-stage burnout could cause the case to fail, particularly when fine-grain investments are involved. The second burnout stage should reach its maximum temperature as prescribed by the manufacturers of the investment and alloy. The alloy manufacturer may suggest a maximum burnout temperature, but this must fall within the limits of the investment. After proper hold time, the case is ready for casting.

Casting

Although casting techniques vary with the types of alloys used and with the various casting systems that are available today, quality control relies heavily on the technician and how much attention is paid to detail. Much has been written about the castability of noble metal alloys as opposed to base metal alloys. It suffices to say that with either alloy, even though a torch can produce excellent results, automatic casting systems such as induc-

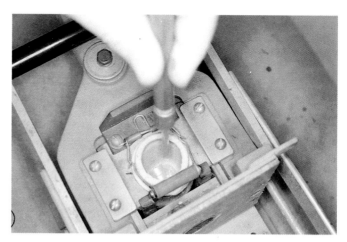

Fig 2-10 Regardless which casting system is used (torch or automatic), attention must be paid to detail; overheating or underheating could bring about an unacceptable casting. The molten metal must be cast at the exact temperature prescribed for it; often it is difficult to visually recognize this. An automatic casting system eliminates the possibility of over- or underheating the alloy. It is designed to initiate casting at a predetermined set temperature. It is especially recommended for casting base metal alloys; their correct casting temperatures are more difficult to recognize than those of the noble metal alloys.

tion are more capable of controlling quality; the element of chance is eliminated. Regardless which method is used, however, the possibility of a faulty casting is greater with base metal alloys.

When comparing base with noble metal alloy, the relatively higher melting temperature and the difficulty in recognizing it makes it vulnerable to both over- and underheating. Overheating will burn out needed ingredients for hardness, strength, and proper coefficient of expansion. Underheating can cause "metal freeze," resulting in a miscast. This is brought about by the inability to recognize the ideal casting temperature or the "slumping" point. This critical temperature is more easily recognized in the noble metal alloys. The higher temperatures required for melting base metals and the narrow safe temperature margin make it more difficult to consistently produce flawless castings (Fig 2-10).

Accurate waxing, spruing, investing, burnout, and casting are essential for acceptable results, especially with base metal alloys. Resistance to flow, need for more sophisticated investments, higher melting temperatures, and need for certain trace elements make casting results of base metal alloys more difficult to predict. Noble metal alloys have been in use longer than base metal alloys, hence there has been more time for improvement. Also, less complicated formulas have made improvement easier. Base metal alloys, in contrast, are more complex in formulation and are relatively new on the market.

Hardness

When referring to hardness of a metal substructure in a porcelain-to-metal system, we refer to wear resistance. When comparing the hardness of noble metal and base metal alloys, the difference between the two is significant. Initially, ceramic golds had the reputation as being the hardest alloy in dentistry. As improvements were made and newer alloys such as the "semiprecious" and base metal alloys were developed, it was found that harder alloys could serve well as a substructure for porcelain, possessing even more advantages than were found in the earlier noble metal alloys. The large array of base metal alloys on the market today shows a tremendous improvement over those developed in the early years of porcelain-to-metal systems and have afforded the dentist and technician a large range to choose from.

The degree of hardness needed in the substructure of a ceramic restoration should be determined by the amount of exposed metal that will be in direct contact with other functional components of the completed restoration. These functional surfaces must be able to withstand any frictional contact that might be applied to it and furthermore should be of equal hardness. The best example of this philosophy is found where a removable partial denture is used in conjunction with a ceramic restoration. Removable partial dentures are designed to obtain maximum retention while distributing minimal stresses equally throughout the entire dental arch.

As mentioned earlier, the prerequisites for a sound metal substructure vary from case to case. In some cases the relatively soft noble metal alloys are sufficient to comply with the needs for function and durability. Other cases require a much harder alloy in order to sustain wear. The dentist must anticipate the potential wear involved and select an alloy that will best resist it. If there is any doubt about the feasibility of the selection, the laboratory staff should be consulted.

Removable Bar Partial Denture (Figs 2-11a and b)

A removable bar partial denture relies on the retention it receives from the bar incorporated into the ceramic restoration. The bar can be located in an edentulous area and has three flat exposed surfaces. Of the three surfaces, two are parallel and perpendicular to the ridge and are the "working" surfaces. They supply the needed retention to the removable partial denture. The two walls must be surveyed and made to be absolutely parallel with the path of insertion. The frictional retention rendered by the bar is directly proportional to the depth of the walls. The success or failure of this type of partial denture depends on the degree of retention supplied by the bar, its longevity, and how well the working surfaces stand up to constant frictional wear. To select a metal substructure that is softer than the alloy to be used for the removable partial denture frame will greatly shorten its longevity. Most removable partial denture frames are constructed with very hard alloys such as chrome-cobalt type materials, therefore the ceramic substructure selection should be a base metal alloy. Its superior hardness (resistance to wear), as compared to noble metal alloys, will greatly withstand the frictional wear placed upon it by its very hard counterpart. To select a noble

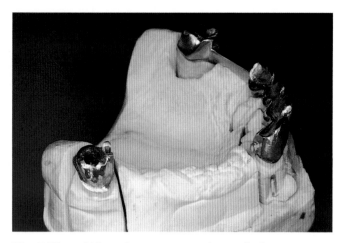

Fig 2-11a When the treatment plan calls for a removable partial denture that relys on a bar for retention, the alloy selection for the permanent partial denture, which will serve as the porcelain substructure, should be one that is capable of withstanding wear. The two parallel walls serve as retention for the removable partial denture and must retain their original dimensions. Because of its hardness and ability to withstand wear, a base metal alloy is recommended.

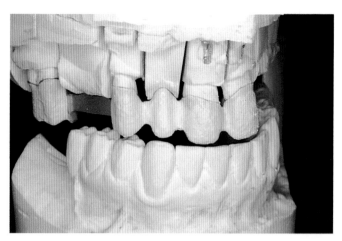

Fig 2-11b Restorations that include a bar depend on it from between 50% to 85% for its retention. The entire restoration, both fixed and removable partial dentures, is constructed according to position and the path of insertion it creates. Each phase of fabrication must conform to its parallel walls in order for the restoration to succeed. Should any of the wall surface wear away, retention could be lost and failure could result. Metal hardness, therefore, is a prime factor in the success or failure of a restoration such as this.

metal alloy for this type of restoration would certainly shorten the life of an otherwise successful restoration.

Dovetails and Semiprecision Attachments (Fig 2-12)

When other means of retention are used for removable partial denture stability, the same reasoning holds true. Dovetails and semiprecision attachments are often called upon to help support the main source of retention such as a bar or precision attachment. Although the retentiveness may not be as critical as the prime source, its ability to withstand wear is just as imperative. Whether it is used alone or in combination with other forms of retention, a base metal alloy should be used.

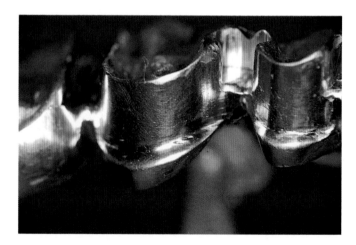

Fig 2-12 Dovetails and semiprecision attachments are often included to act as support for the prime source of retention. It is just as important for this support to be hard enough to resist wear. Should retention be lost because of abrasion by the removable partial denture, failure could result.

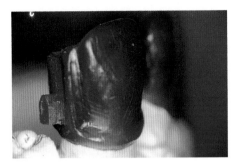

Fig 2-13a

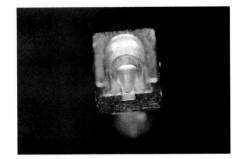

Fig 2-13b

Fig 2-13a Precision attachments are often responsible for much of the retention found in a fixed-removable combination restoration. Their sharp angles and parallel walls are required for this retention. If, during treatment planning, it is found that an abnormal amount of stress is going to be placed on the attachment and a question is raised as to its ability to resist wear, it is advisable to duplicate its fixed component and incorporate it into the base metal casting. This will ensure that the abnormal stresses applied to it will not effect its retention.

Fig 2-13b There is less concern needed for the section of the precision attachment that is placed into the removable partial denture. Should there be retention loss because of wear, the attachment can usually be replaced with little difficulty; in most restorations it is simply luted to the removable frame with acrylic resin.

Precision Attachments (Figs 2-13a and b)

Precision attachments can be used alone or in conjunction with other sources of retention. Regardless which type of attachment is used, there will always be some degree of wear in either or both sections of the attachment. One section in the removable partial denture is usually luted into the acrylic resin, making it easier to replace. The other section in the permanent restoration is either soldered or cast to it, making it almost impossible to replace. For this reason, the section located in the fixed restoration should be slightly harder than the section luted to the removable partial denture. One method for accomplishing this is to duplicate this section and cast it with the metal substructure using a base metal alloy. This will ensure the integrity of the sharp angles and prevent wear from occurring to the walls of the attachment, maintaining maximum retention. If wear occurs in the section embedded in the removable partial denture, the embedded section can be replaced quite easily with assurance that the case is redeemable.

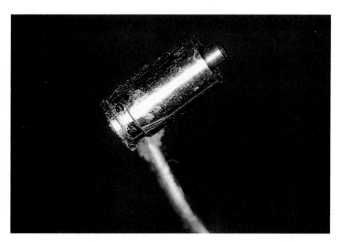

Fig 2-14a The "Tach-Ez" is a typical plunger-type attachment that depends on a dimple placed into the frame of the fixed partial denture for retention. The plunger is forced into the dimple with a spring found in the attachment housing. When the plunger is engaged into the dimple, the removable partial denture is kept firmly in place. This attachment works well alone or in conjunction with other retentive sources in the restoration. The plunger is made from a hard metal alloy and is capable of wearing away any metal surface it glides over that might be softer than the alloy it is composed of.

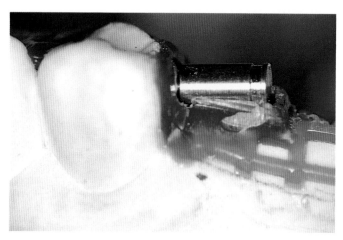

Fig 2-14b A cradle is waxed into the removable partial denture frame. The housing is attached to the cast partial frame with self-curing acrylic resin before setting up the teeth. Upon completion of acrylic resin processing, the attachment housing becomes part of the removable partial denture. The cast cradle and the processed acrylic resin prevent movement and help maintain constant pressure against the fixed restoration. Removal and replacement of the attachment are simple.

Most plunger-type attachments (Figs 2-14a to d) depend on retention derived from a dimple placed into an exposed surface on the metal substructure of the ceramic restoration. The dimple is ground into the framework after the removable partial frame is cast and prepared for incorporating the attachment into it. In cases such as this, the harder base metal alloy will provide a longer life expectancy with less chance of wear than the softer noble metal alloy. The dimple must maintain its dimensions; it provides the sole retention for the plunger-type attachment. If the plunger forms a wear pattern on the working wall of the framework, the case could fail because of loss of retention. This can be prevented by prescribing a base metal alloy rather than a noble metal alloy.

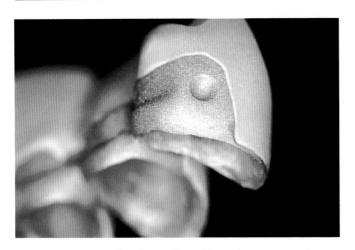

Fig 2-14c The dimple is placed into the cast metal substructure upon completion of porcelain fabrication. The path that the plunger takes over the surface of the casting must be wear resistant. Wear to any degree in this area will cause retention loss to the removable partial denture. The chances of a wear pattern being formed are much greater in a precious metal alloy than in a base metal alloy. In fact, the base metal alloy will show no wear and therefore is the best selection for a porcelain metal substructure when used in conjunction with a plunger-type attachment.

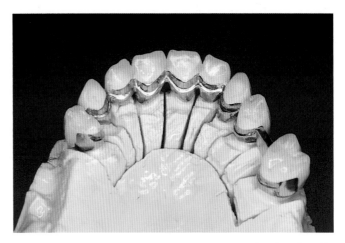

Fig 2-14d The dimples will be placed on the distal walls of the maxillary first premolar and left first molar. In this case, the plunger-type attachment has assistance from the bar and milled lingual area. The distal retention of the removable partial denture will depend greatly on its ability to maintain its path of insertion over the distal walls that must be free of wear. The plunger's path of insertion must be parallel with all other surfaces in contact with the removable partial frame (ie, the bar and milled lingual surfaces).

Milled Restorations (Figs 2-15a to c)

A milled removable partial denture, when used with a well-engineered porcelain-to-metal substructure, can be very advantageous when constructing a functionally sound restoration. It not only assists in distributing the occlusal load evenly over the entire arch, it also contributes to better esthetics in that in most cases, it eliminates the need for clasps.

Two requirements needed for milling to succeed are: (1) well-designed, scalloped-type, contoured walls on the ceramic metal framework that are high enough for retention and parallel with the path of insertion, and (2) wear-resistant walls. Regardless of how well the walls are surveyed and made parallel for maximum retention of the removable partial denture, the slightest wearing away of the wall surfaces will cause the restoration to fail. For this reason, when a hard frame for a removable partial denture (chrome-cobalt) is used, it is imperative to use an alloy for the ceramic metal framework that is close to the same hardness. Noble metal alloys cannot qualify as a durable material in this situation hence a base metal alloy should be considered. The closer the hardness match between the permanent and removable metal framework, the less wearing away there will be and thus the less chance of failure. If loss of retention occurs because of wear, the most logical approach would be to construct a new removable partial denture.

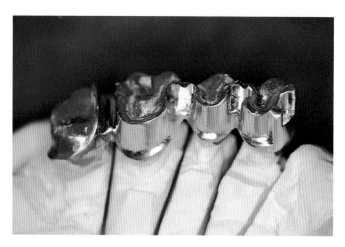

Fig 2-15a An accurately milled porcelain substructure can supply adequate retention for a removable partial denture. Proper design is important (ie, parallel walls that are high enough to furnish required surface area and constructed to coordinate with other retentive facilities in the restoration). Alloy selection, however, is just as important because the slightest surface wear to the metal substructure could forfeit enough retention to render the restoration useless. For this reason the alloy should be at least as hard as the removable partial denture frame.

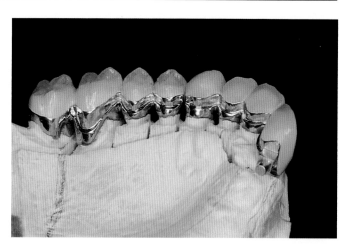

Fig 2-15b A milled metal substructure can contribute greatly to the esthetic value of the restoration. It helps distribute the load uniformly throughout while supplying retention without the need of unsightly clasps. A well-engineered, milled metal substructure, with sufficient hardness, can be efficient with the aid of a single precision attachment. The alloy hardness should correspond with the attachment and both should be wear resistant.

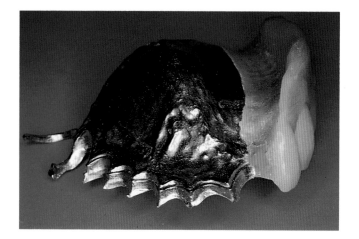

Fig 2-15c The scalloped design in the framework of the removable partial denture is contoured to fit snugly in the milled area of the metal substructure of the fixed partial denture. Their surfaces function together to create retention. The hard alloy (chrome-cobalt derivative) of the partial denture frame will wear away the surface of a precious metal alloy. Some semiprecious alloys will survive this friction, but when in doubt during planning and alloy selection, a base metal alloy should be considered.

Margins and Fine Bevels (Fig 2-16)

Perhaps the most vulnerable area of the restoration is the margin, especially a beveled margin. Even though all of the above requirements for hardness may be met in a restoration exhibiting excellent fit and function, if the fine beveled margin is damaged or polished away, the restoration would obviously be unacceptable. Care must be taken, therefore, to retain the integrity of these finely beveled margins that are responsible for a superior seal. The relatively soft noble metal alloy stands a better chance of being damaged or worn away during the polishing phase than the much harder base metal alloy. During case planning, if the trimmed dies show extremely fine beveled margins (especially on multiunit cases where these margins are in close proximity and proper finishing and polishing could be difficult), a base metal alloy should be considered for the metal substructure. Fine beveled margins can be waxed to a sharp edge with little danger of miscast, resulting in hard margins, eliminating any possibility of damage or wear during finishing and polishing.

Summary

During case planning, it is important to recognize when alloy hardness will play an important role in the success of the restoration. Removable partial dentures are especially prone to failure if an alloy with insufficient hardness is selected for the ceramic substructure. The greater the hardness, the less chance of surface wear. It is obvious, therefore, that when selecting an alloy for the metal substructure in cases that require wear resistance, a base metal alloy should be chosen over a noble metal alloy.

Strength

The strength of base metal alloy, as with its hardness, is superior to that of noble metal alloy. In thin

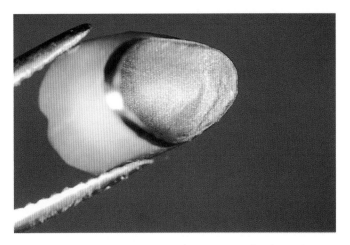

Fig 2-16 A restoration may function perfectly and meet all esthetic requirements yet may be unacceptable because the finely beveled margin was worn away during finishing and polishing. The possibility of wearing away a beveled margin in a precious metal alloy restoration is much greater than in a restoration using an alloy with sufficient hardness to maintain a fine knife edge during polishing.

areas of a restoration that depend almost entirely on the strength of the metal substructure, base metal alloy should be considered. Thin metal substructure and margins, thin supporting walls for dovetails, semiprecision attachments, and interlocks require strength to withstand movement and bending.

On multiunit restorations, often there is insufficient room for adequate interproximal connections. This may be the fault of a close bite or lack of room for gingival tissue. Skimpy metal connections require the strength of an alloy that will not distort during porcelain fabrication or fracture during mastication. For this reason, base metal alloy should be considered because its strength is several times greater than that of noble metal alloy, and the chances of distortion during porcelain fabrication or fracture during mastication are slim. Noble metal alloy would be questionable (Figs 2-17 to 2-19).

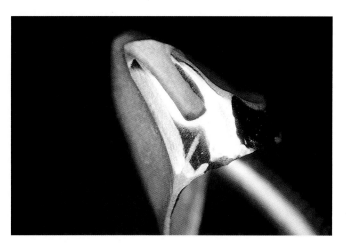

Fig 2-17 Thin walls of the female portion of a dovetail connection must be capable of withstanding heavy loads and must maintain their integrity during functional occlusion. Often it is impossible to supply required thickness in order for a noble metal alloy to absorb these stresses with no distortion. A very thin-walled section of a dovetail can, however, withstand these stresses when a base metal alloy is used.

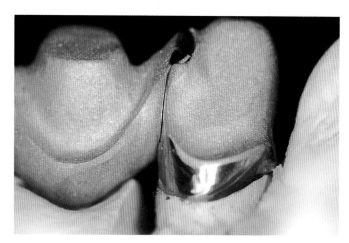

Fig 2-18 Dovetail connections, whether cemented or free, should have very little or no tolerance in order to function properly. They are used primarily where the path of insertion has created a problem for seating. When periodontal problems are involved and rigidity is required to stabilize otherwise mobile teeth, the dovetailed connection is important for maintaining this rigidity.

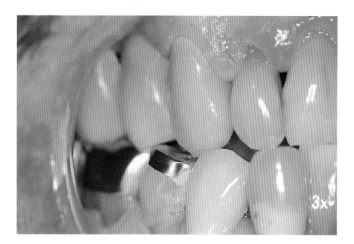

Fig 2-19 Seated three-unit dovetailed restoration. In situations that involve malocclusion, such as this, a restoration must be capable of sustaining excessive forces. The thin-walled dovetail attachment must be strong enough to resist distortion and breakage. A base metal alloy will supply the needed strength in ultra-thin-walled attachments that cannot be obtained with noble metal alloy.

The success and longevity of a restoration may rely entirely on the strength of the metal substructure in certain strategic areas.

Tissue and Wear

When selecting the best suited alloy for a ceramic substructure, oral health must also be taken into account. Two very important health factors that are directly related to the metal substructure are (1) periodontal tissue surrounding the tooth root and (2) periodontal wear to the incisal or occlusal surfaces that are in function with the ceramic restoration.

Periodontal Tissue Abuse

One theory that deals with periodontal tissue suggests that certain occluding materials could promote periodontal tissue destruction by transferring occlusal stresses to that area of the tooth. This theory contends that the degree of stress is directly proportional to the hardness of the material. Occluding materials in increasing order of hardness are: (1) acrylic resin, (2) noble metal alloy, (3) dental porcelain, and (4) base metal alloy. The theory is based on the fact that softer materials tend to absorb or cushion most of the occlusal stresses whereas harder materials tend to transfer stresses. It is also a fact that in an ideal environment, where a perfectly equilibrated occlusion is in evidence, the load is distributed evenly throughout the entire arch, thus eliminating excessive stress in any one area. This is not always the circumstance; however, there are some situations where it is impossible to obtain ideal occlusion. When periodontal health is in question and a "cushion effect" is needed, the much softer noble metal alloy should be selected rather than base metal alloy (Fig 2-20). Further, the metal substructure should be designed such that the occluding surface functions with the opposing dentition to afford maximum protection. For example, noble metal alloy exposed on the lingual surface of the maxillary six anterior restorations will help cushion both the maxillary and mandibular anterior regions while lingual cusps formed in noble metal alloy will help cushion the maxillary and mandibular posterior regions. The very hard base metal alloys cannot offer this protection and should be ruled out where periodontal tissue health is a concern.

Incisal and Occlusal Wear

Concern should also be directed toward incisal and occlusal wear to dentition that opposes the seated restoration. Close evaluation of mounted diagnostic models during case planning will show potential wear patterns and should clearly indicate if wear to opposing dentition will be a concern. When selecting a metal substructure for restorations involving a potential wear problem to

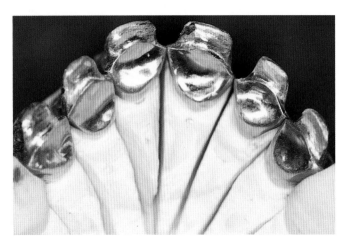

Fig 2-20 When there is concern for surrounding periodontal tissue and possible wear to occluding dentition, a noble metal alloy should be considered for the substructure. Compared to a base metal alloy, a noble metal alloy is relatively soft and could act as a cushion to the periodontal tissue and opposing dentition. The "cushion effect" is more pronounced when metal is exposed to contact with the opposing dentition. Noble metal alloy will tend to wear and give slightly, rather than transmit all of the forces to the supporting periodontal tissue.

opposing dentition, consider noble metal alloy with a high-gold content. When the opposing dentition occludes with the surface of the relatively soft high-gold content metal, wear to the dentition will be minimal. Occluding with base metal, however, could cause excessive wear. Thus, noble metal alloy is the logical choice when wear is a concern.

Veneer Advantage

The strength of base metal alloys far surpass that of noble metal alloys. In order to justify its use, maintaining enough strength to withstand distortion and breakage, a noble metal alloy substructure must be bulkier in all areas, including the veneering surfaces of the restoration (Fig 2-21). A minimum thickness of 0.3 mm of noble metal alloy

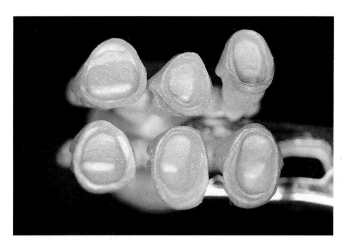

Fig 2-21 This noble metal alloy casting shows the needed thickness when used as a substructure to support porcelain. Note the bulky margins and the overall "sluggish" appearance. For proper support free of warpage and fracture, minimum thickness throughout should be 0.3 mm. This could be troublesome, especially in an anterior restoration with an ultra-thin labial veneer. The bulky metal substructure takes up room that could otherwise be occupied with porcelain.

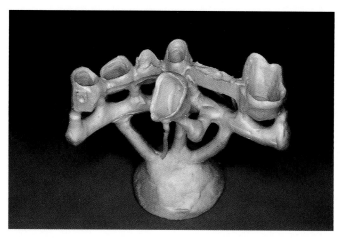

Fig 2-22 This base metal alloy casting shows thin-walled and well-defined margins. Substructures fabricated with base metal alloy can be as thin as 0.1 mm and can withstand any incisal or occlusal force directed to it without distortion or fracture. This makes available to the ceramist more labial and buccal thickness for porcelain. It promotes opportunity for better color and more vitality to the restoration than could be obtained in a thinner veneer using noble metal alloy as the substructure.

in the veneer wall is required to establish sufficient strength to support porcelain, as compared to the 0.1 mm thickness needed for a base metal alloy substructure (Fig 2-22). Anterior restorations that are critical for esthetic reasons depend greatly on an adequate thickness of porcelain. The additional 0.2 mm of porcelain made available when using a base metal alloy substructure could make a difference in the esthetic result of the restoration. In such cases, selecting base metal alloy for the substructure would be a definite advantage.

Prefabrication Connection

The most vulnerable area in any multiple-unit restoration is the connection between each unit. Choosing the proper connecting method is critical for a successful restoration. In order to select the best connection method for any given restoration,

several factors must be considered: (1) the alloy to be used in the restoration, (2) the amount of area allotted for the connection, (3) load distribution (pontics, precision attachments, etc), and (4) abnormalities in occlusion.

There are several prefabrication connection methods available to choose from: (1) cast connections, (2) unsoldered dovetails, (3) soldered dovetails, and (4) prefabrication soldered connections. Each has advantages and disadvantages. The strongest is the cast connection (Fig 2-23). When comparing noble metal with base metal alloy, the base metal connection is stronger. The next strongest connection is the dovetail type using solid parent metal interproximally (Fig 2-24). The least desirable is the prefabrication soldered connection; its biggest disadvantage is the potential distortion that occurs during porcelain fabrication. The high temperature required to fabricate porcelain has the capacity to distort the

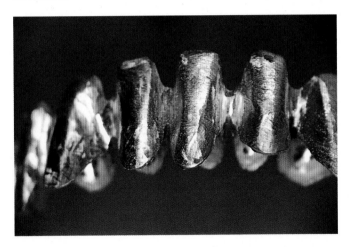

Fig 2-23 Cast connections provide maximum interproximal strength for any given alloy, as opposed to prefabricated soldered connections that are somewhat weaker and prone to warpage during porcelain application. The required interproximal metal thickness will depend on the alloy; it is directly proportional to the gold content of the alloy, base metal connections being much stronger than noble metal alloy.

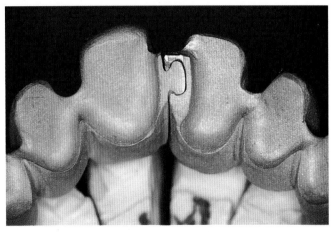

Fig 2-24 Soldered or unsoldered dovetailed connections are strong and can help solve problems that sometimes plague metal substructures. Where path of insertion problems and need for segment castings are involved in a restoration, dovetailing can be used with complete assurance that the connection will have adequate strength. (With path of insertion problems, the dovetails are left unsoldered; otherwise, single castings can be soldered after porcelain fabrication.)

restoration at the soldered connections. After only several firings, microscopic observation shows enough distortion in most cases to prevent perfect seating. Without the use of a microscope, many distortions go unnoticed, allowing restorations to be seated with less than a perfect fit.

Another complication associated with prefabrication soldered connections occurs by introducing two foreign alloys into the restoration: the solder and the resulting alloy formed by the solder and parent metal at the area immediate to the connection. The coefficient of expansion in this area becomes questionable and could cause the porcelain over the connection to "pull away" and fracture.

Although prefabrication soldering is not recommended for either the noble or base metal alloys, noble metal alloys exhibit slightly more success. The nature of the noble metal alloy, ie, its lower melting point and uncomplicated chemical formula, gives it a slight edge over base metal alloy. The higher melting temperatures required for base metal alloys and their susceptibility to heavy oxidation deposits make it difficult to obtain even a mediocre solder connection. The need for heavy concentrations of flux to help curb oxidation adds to the dilemma because flux is often responsible for porous connections, which in turn weaken the connections and could also create bubbling, fracturing, and possibly porcelain veneer separation.

Alternatives to Prefabrication Soldering

The two best alternatives to prefabrication soldering noble metal alloys are (1) multiunit casting with solid cast connections and (2) postfabrication soldered connections.

The best alternatives to prefabrication soldering base metal alloys are multiunit casting (postfabrication soldered connections are not consistently acceptable in the case of base metal alloys), and Dr Peter Weiss's technique for double casting. Weiss's technique has proven to be of great value in repairing base metal miscasts before porcelain fabrication. The technique is an alternative to reconstructing a restoration that has been miscast resulting in an incomplete or ill-fitting casting.

An incomplete base metal casting can result from (1) an ultrathin wax pattern that hinders the flow of molten metal, (2) improper spruing (gauge and location), (3) underheated casting ring, (4) insufficient heat to melt the alloy for proper flow, and (5) investment breakdown.

With an ill-fitting multiple-unit restoration caused by distortion, each die fits perfectly into its casting but the restoration as a unit does not seat perfectly. This usually indicates a fault in spruing or possible pattern disruption while removing the wax pattern from the master model. It occurs quite often when large pontics are involved. Results such as this are unacceptable.

A minor casting flaw could mean wasted time and labor with a possible profit loss. Probably the most frustrating situation is a multiple-unit distorted casting. Even the most quality-oriented laboratory experiences this, and if a method is not devised to redeem these miscasts and distorted castings, remakes could become very costly.

Double-casting techniques. One such method used successfully to repair and restore an unacceptable metal substructure is the double casting technique devised by Weiss. It entails repairing the flaw by recasting to the original metal substructure. Although this technique is prescribed primarily for base metal alloys, it has also been known to be successful when used in conjunction with noble metal alloys. This technique has virtually no limits in that it is useful in repairing minor and major miscasts, replacing one or more individual castings to a full splint, and reorienting a distorted splint to the master model. This technique can also be used to attach interproximally before porcelain application.

The most significant feature in this technique is its physical attachment, rather than chemical bond. The high oxidation factor associated with all base metal alloys prevents a chemical union when this double casting system is used. Success, therefore, rests entirely on a physical connection and depends greatly on how the metal is prepared.

Metal preparation. Minor incomplete casting (single wall) (Figs 2-25a to c): Proper metal framework preparation to accept the second casting is critical. The technique requires that there be sufficient surface area to contact the new metal and sufficient nonparallel dovetailing to lock it in place. This is accomplished with a barrel-shaped carbide bur used to prepare the wall so that it develops as much surface area as possible that is angled in as many directions as possible.

Major miscast (single wall with wax pattern) (Figs 2-26a to c): A miscast of a more serious nature can also be repaired using this technique. The miscast may be such that a completely new wax pattern must be made and incorporated into the second casting. This could involve one or several newly waxed patterns, an important factor being accurate seating of the patterns and original casting to achieve perfect alignment. The original casting is prepared with a dovetail, using as much surface area as possible. The attachment area depends mainly on the available proximal surface of the casting to which the connection will be made. If no interproximal area is available, the dovetail can be cut into the crown, as would be done for an incomplete casting. When a pontic is to be part of the cast connection, there is no question as to the amount of available surface area, and the pontics add greatly to the possibility of a successful repair. The dovetail can be cut deep and angled in several directions, ensuring a securely locked-in connection.

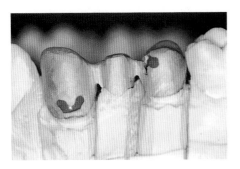

Fig 2-25a

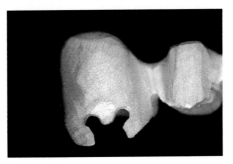

Fig 2-25b

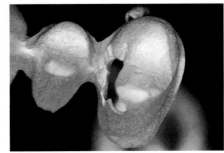

Fig 2-25c

Fig 2-25a   Minor miscasts occur occasionally in the laboratory and can be attributed to a thin wax pattern, improper spruing, insufficiently heated investment, and/or alloy and investment breakdown. The two flaws in this casting were caused by investment breakdown; pieces of investment lodged in the labial margin of the maxillary right canine and the mesiobucco-occlusal surface of the second premolar. Rather than reconstruct the restoration or attempt to repair with solder (preporcelain fabrication soldering technique), the double casting technique could be used.

Fig 2-25b   Preparing the original casting to accept new alloy is very important in that bonding is physical, not chemical, due to the oxidation that takes place over the surface of the original casting. For this reason, the bonding surface must be dovetailed in several different directions so that a physical bond will occur, securing the new casting in place. One requirement for a successful second casting is that the dovetailed walls of the casting are thick enough (approximately 0.2 mm) to establish a physical grip. If this minimum thickness is not available, it is advisable to rewax the units and recast.

Fig 2-25c   The walls of posterior castings are usually thick enough for dovetailing so that a secure physical bond is certain. In posterior areas that are subjected to great forces, the miscast area should be widened and prepared so that more surface area is obtained for better retention. This also permits more dovetailing, which lends to a better physical bond.

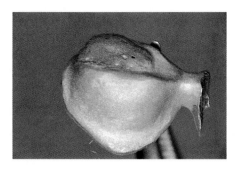

Fig 2-26a

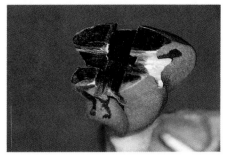

Fig 2-26b

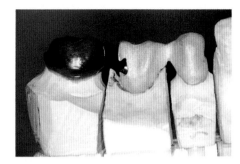

Fig 2-26c

Fig 2-26a   A major miscast will necessitate removal of the unit or units from the original casting and preparation of adjacent units to accept the second casting. An ill-fitting unit or one with excessive porosity could be considered a major miscast. A miscast with walls too thin to dovetail would also be reason enough to replace it completely.

Fig 2-26b   When replacing the entire unit, the adjacent unit must be prepared with maximum surface area for a satisfactory connection. This type of repair must be able to withstand stronger forces than are found on a minor repair, especially in the posterior region. When a pontic is the adjacent unit, dovetailing is a simple matter because the pontic thickness is more than enough to provide abundant surface area for a superior physical bond.

Fig 2-26c   A major miscast usually requires completely rewaxing the unit or units involved. Care must be taken to seat the die perfectly into its original position on the master working model. The master working model should be mounted back onto the articulator, making sure the functional aspects of the restoration are satisfied. The second waxing should correct the problem that brought about the miscast (ie, correct wax thickness and proper sprue placement with possible venting).

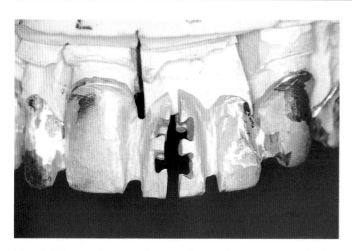

Fig 2-27a When each unit of a multiunit casting fits its die perfectly but the full casting does not seat completely, the probable reason is distortion. This could be brought about during waxing, spruing, investing, and/or casting. Heavy pontics in a restoration is a major cause of distortion. Usually a single separation is sufficient; however, in some cases several separations may be necessary. A logical initial separation would be in the pontic. Both sections of the pontic are dovetailed, exposing as much surface area as possible.

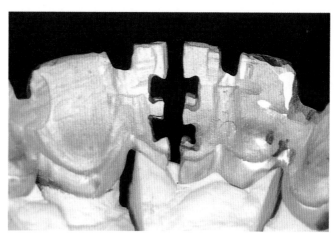

Fig 2-27b After the initial separation, the two halves of the multiunit substructure are placed back onto the master working model and checked with a microscope, both buccally and lingually, for fit and seating. Separations can also be made interproximally or in any cast unit. It seldom takes more than one slice. If a single separation does not accomplish this, another should be made and reevaluated.

Frame distortion (double wall connection) (Figs 2-27a and b): In a multiunit casting, when each casting fits perfectly into its respective die and the path of insertion is parallel but the entire unit does not seat properly, the probable reason is a distortion in the metal frame. Frame distortion is unacceptable and the restoration must be either reconstructed or corrected. Reconstruction could be costly, whereas correction is relatively inexpensive.

The first step in repairing a distorted frame is to locate the pivot point of the distortion. This will require either bisecting a casting, interproximal connection, or pontic. Regardless where the separation is made, the same rule prevails: secure as much surface area as possible with maximum unparallelism. This may mean cutting in several locations.

Cases involving large pontics are exceptionally vulnerable to distortion. When this occurs, the pontic is bisected and dovetails are cut into both walls. The thick unparallel walls will serve well as a base for the second casting with assurance the connections will be strong with no fear of separation.

Waxing. *Minor incomplete casting (single wall) (Figs 2-28a to d):* In the case of an incomplete casting, it is essential that all units involved be seated back on the master model perfectly before any attempt is made to repair the miscast. Where margins are involved, extra care must be taken to accurately replace in wax the area that was incomplete. If the casting is not perfectly seated on the master model, a wax replacement will be inaccurate, resulting in an ill-fitting restoration. After adapting wax to the miscast area, a thin wax overlap is made in the immediate area to ensure a complete physical connection.

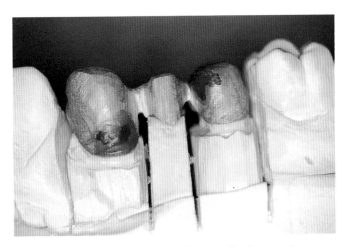

Fig 2-28a After seating the dies perfectly into the master working model and lubricating them, the casting is placed onto the dies and the flaws are waxed. When flowing wax to metal, care must be taken to heat the wax sufficiently so that it clings to the cool metal. Otherwise it could be repelled by the metal before it forms a secure bond.

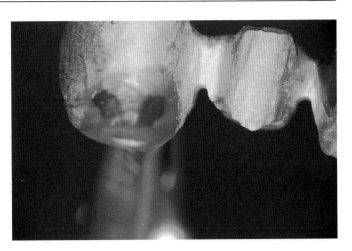

Fig 2-28b A thin overlay of wax is placed onto the metal to ensure a complete casting. The thin metal overlay will not bond to the original casting because of oxidation; this overlay will be ground away during metal finishing. If the dies are properly lubricated, the wax should be released with no flaws or distortion. In marginal miscasts such as this, it is advisable to overbuild slightly.

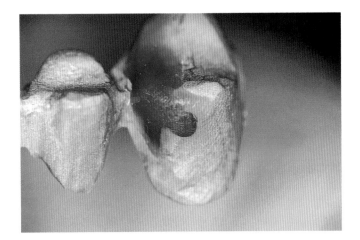

Fig 2-28c Occlusal flaws should also be overwaxed slightly; it should be thick enough so that the second casting will be able to support occlusal forces placed upon it. (Note the thin wax overlay.) Care should be taken not to incorporate the same condition that caused the miscast in the original casting.

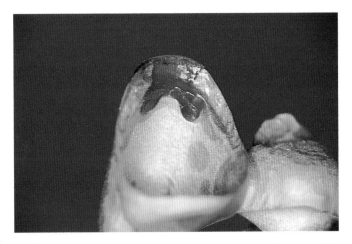

Fig 2-28d The casting should be examined internally, verifying sharp margins and a wax-to-metal bond. A microscope will reveal waxing flaws and gaps between wax and metal if they exist. The wax should be a perfect negative reproduction of the die's surface to ensure a well-sealed finished casting.

Major miscast (single wall with wax pattern) (Fig 2-29): A miscast that includes one or more full units will require a complete rewaxing, which could mean having to articulate and establish proper occlusion and function. If the involved unit or units are full-metal cast units, required occlusion and function must be carved into the wax pasterns and should be completed before attaching them to the original casting. If the units require a porcelain veneer, an even thickness of wax is cut back (1 mm) to permit room for eventual porcelain application.

Upon completing the wax pattern, the margins are sealed and the dies are seated perfectly into the master model, making sure the patterns and original casting are in proper alignment. The waxed units are then luted together and waxed into the dovetailed original casting. Care must be taken to flow the wax well into the dovetail, adapting it completely over the entire prepared wall to ensure a strong physical bond. A thin layer of wax is overlapped onto the original casting to ensure a complete casting.

Frame distortion: The most important factor is to precisely seat the restoration onto the master model before luting with wax. With the distorted frame repair there is no concern for replacing lost margins; the main concern is that each cut section fit onto the master model, completely eliminating any sign of "rocking." Once this is accomplished, the same rules for waxing apply as for any other repair. Flow wax into the dovetail making sure none of the walls are exposed; create a thin overlap to ensure a complete casting. There is no need to overwax the connection unless additional strength is needed. Overbuilding means extra grinding after casting, which results in added expense and time spent.

Spruing, investing, burnout and casting.

Spruing (Figs 2-30a to d): Two types of spruing are required in this technique — direct and support. Any addition must be sprued directly from the metal reservoir, whether it be a full crown wax pattern or a mere sliver of margin. Venting may be used to

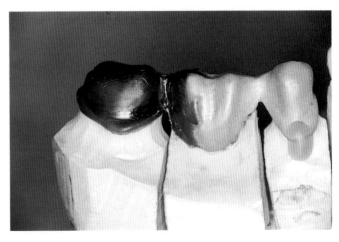

Fig 2-29 In a major miscast where one or more units must be fully rewaxed, care must be taken to properly position these newly waxed units before waxing into the dovetailed adjacent unit. Also, interproximal waxed connections must be heavy enough to supply maximum strength to the new casting.

ensure a complete casting by permitting the escape of gases. Support sprues are added to hold the casting in place during investing. These sprues also originate at the metal source and extend to areas of the original casting. Oxidation during wax burnout will prevent an attachment between the supporting sprue and casting, its only purpose being support during investing. After firmly attaching the sprues (direct and support) and possible vents, debubblizer is applied and the case is made ready for investing.

Investing: Follow exact investing procedure prescribed by the manufacturer of the investment. The same investment, powder:liquid ratio, and mixing time, are used as were used for the original casting. After setting, the case is ready for burnout and casting.

Burnout and casting: The burnout and casting procedures are also the same as for the original casting, using identical time and temperature formulas. The oxidation that takes place during wax

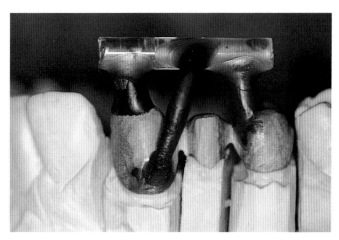

Fig 2-30a Direct spruing is made from a runner bar to the newly waxed areas. Care must be taken not to distort the wax in these areas when attaching the sprue. Sprues and attachments should be rounded and smooth so the molten metal will flow freely; this lessens the possibility of investment particles breaking off and causing further complications. Along with the feeder sprue, at least one support sprue is necessary to hold the original casting stationary during investing (incisal of canine).

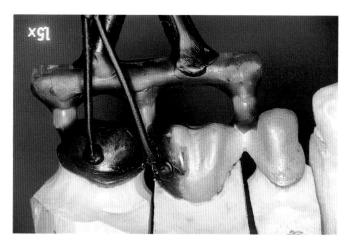

Fig 2-30b The amount of spruing required will vary, depending on the extent of the repair (ie, a fully waxed unit may need several sprues). Venting can also be used to permit the escape of heat and gases during casting procedures. Vents are attached to both thin and bulky areas (buccal surface of molar and pontic dovetail). Note support sprue at interproximal of pontic and premolar.

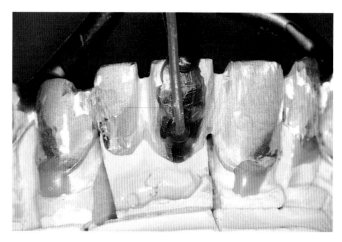

Fig 2-30c Large restorations require several support sprues, especially one such as this where the casting is completely separated and dovetailed (maxillary left central pontic). Note the entire casting is held in place with sticky wax during waxing and spruing. Also, note a vent is attached to the waxed dovetailed area.

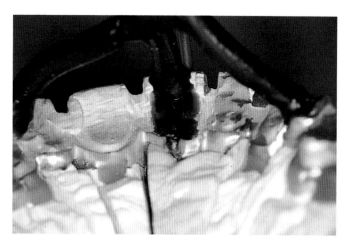

Fig 2-30d Flow direction of the molten alloy is important and will depend on wax thickness and type of repair. In this casting, which has a relatively thick wax connection and a complex dovetailed pattern with a large surface area, the sprue is placed lingually so the alloy can flow directly into the dovetail, linguolabially rather than incisogingivally. As the alloy enters lingually, the heat and gases escape labially through a vent.

burnout prevents a chemical bond during casting, thus making a physical bond at the dovetail connection.

Dressing metal (preparing for porcelain): After casting, the ring is allowed to bench cool. Upon deflasking, the direct sprues and vents are cut off (supporting sprues are not attached due to oxidation) and the metal substructure is prepared for porcelain application.

The thin metal flash is ground flush with the newly cast metal and is contoured to conform with the original substructure design. Spraying with aluminum oxide (50 μm) and cleansing with steam will assure a sterile environment for porcelain application. Normal veneering procedures are rendered with no need for alteration. If all requirements are fulfilled, the completed restoration should be of excellent quality with no compromise in strength or esthetic value (Figs 2-31 to 2-36).

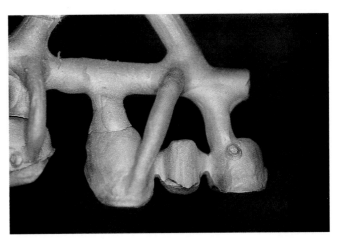

Fig 2-31 Casting after deflasking shows two areas repaired with the double-casting technique. Note the feeder sprues held in place at the dovetailed areas (canine labial margin and premolar bucco-occlusal), whereas the support sprue is unattached due to oxidation (incisal edge of canine).

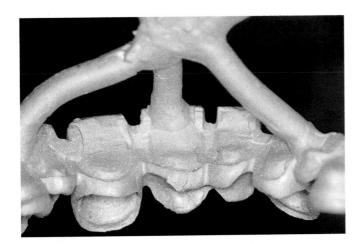

Fig 2-32 Dovetailed area in maxillary left central incisor pontic is completely filled with new alloy, joining together the two halves of the metal substructure. Individual units can be joined together in the same manner by dovetailing interproximally; that is, units in a full-arch restoration can be cast individually or in segments and splinted together using the double-casting technique with dovetailed connections. This produces a stronger restoration with less complications than found in a prefabrication soldering procedure.

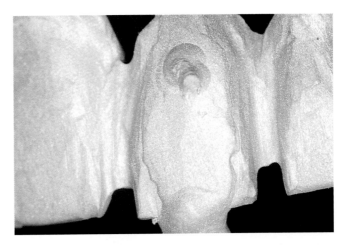

Fig 2-33 Magnified labial view of maxillary left central incisor showing dense second casting into dovetailed area. Note the thin metal overlap that will be ground away during metal finishing. This technique is capable of producing a connection almost as strong as a solid casting and can be used in almost every repair and unit connection before porcelain application.

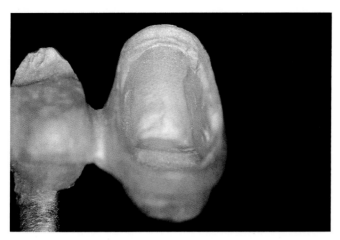

Fig 2-34 The inside of the maxillary second premolar shows the repaired area (bucco-occlusal). To repair this unit with solder would produce a weakened wall with possible complications during porcelain fabrication, such as coefficient of expansion mismatch and/or improper oxidation for bonding. The time saved in not having to reconstruct the entire substructure makes it worth the effort to use the double-casting technique for repairs such as this.

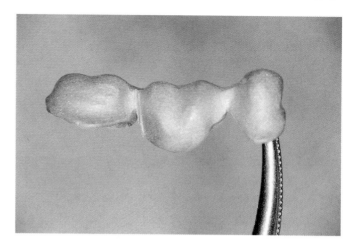

Fig 2-35 Double-cast, three-unit substructure, dressed down and ready for porcelain application. The dovetailed molar pontic supplies excellent connection with the newly cast second molar. The interproximal strength is much greater than could be obtained with solder. The dovetailed connection is undetectable. When properly executed this technique can supply the strength necessary for the substructure to withstand all occlusal forces directed to it.

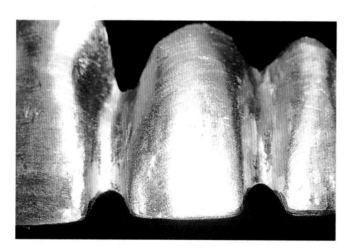

Fig 2-36 Dovetailed maxillary left central incisor pontic holding together a multiunit substructure. The thin metal overlap has been ground away during metal finishing, revealing an undetectable connection. In large multiunit restorations such as this, the double-casting technique could save much time and expense in lieu of redoing the entire substructure. A prefabrication soldered connection in this case, as in most, would be inferior in strength with potential distortion during porcelain fabrication.

Conclusion

Prefabrication soldered connections should *not* be considered a viable alternative to cast connections. This is especially true where base metal alloy is concerned. Even though noble metal alloys have better qualifications for such a connection than do base metal alloys, neither show results that could be considered acceptable for strength and function.

Two alternatives to a prefabrication soldered connection are (1) a multiple unit casting that produces the strongest connection for any given alloy which is free from distortion during porcelain fabrication, and (2) the Weiss double-casting method, which eliminates the need for soldering and produces physical connections that are equal to the strength and function qualities of a cast connection.

The Weiss double-casting method produces a physical connection rather than chemical due to the oxidation layer that is developed during wax burnout. This technique is used successfully in repairing a miscast, adding units to a previously cast metal substructure, and joining two or more metal sections. When properly performed, this technique produces excellent results and is a reliable alternative to prefabrication soldered connection.

Postfabrication Soldered Connection

Postfabrication soldered connections are the connections made between individual units after porcelain fabrication has been completed. In contrast with prefabrication soldered connections, the postfabrication soldered connections are very dependable, especially when used in conjunction with noble metal alloys. In spite of improvements made in recent years, postfabrication soldered connections between base metal units are not nearly as reliable as those made using noble metal. Even well-fluxed walls at times cannot prevent oxidation from occurring during soldering. This, coupled with flux inclusion into the soldered connection, attributes to a weak union with danger of fracture.

Advantages

When noble metal alloys are used there are several advantages in employing postfabrication soldering as a means for connecting individual units.

Individuality: In cases where it is difficult to obtain natural, individual appearing restorations in a multiple-unit casting, postsoldering the units gives the technician an opportunity to contour each unit separately, thus contributing to a more esthetic restoration.

Strength and stability: The strength and stability of a postsoldered connection is maintained primarily because of relatively lower temperatures required for solder flow, with no concern for oxidation when used with nobel metal alloy. Flux is unnecessary, therefore the possibility of porous weak connections is lessened. Also, the connections will not have to withstand several firings during porcelain fabrication, which ensures their stability.

Metal finishing: Having the opportunity to finish the metal of each unit separately gives the technician easier access to otherwise difficult areas to reach. It also lessens the possibility of polishing away finely beveled margins that are often included in a restoration to prevent leakage.

Procedure

Postsoldering porcelain fabricated units with a noble metal substructure is uncomplicated and predictable. A method that has proven successful uses a horizontal porcelain furnace in conjunction with a torch.

After the units have been glazed and the metal has been rubber wheeled to a dull smooth finish, each unit is placed back onto the master model. Each porcelain unit must be contoured so that a fine hairline space separates them. The separation must be enough to allow for expansion during soldering but narrow enough to hide underlying solder. The units are then luted together with sticky wax and a metal bar is attached to add more support and prevent distortion. After the wax has been completely hardened, the luted units are lifted from the model and invested with low-temperature soldering investment, leaving the porcelain exposed. High-temperature investments should not be used; binders are not completely burned off at soldering temperatures and will settle on the surface of the porcelain, leaving a spotty glaze. After the investment has set up completely, the wax is eliminated with boiling water, the investment is trimmed, and sluice ways are cut to each separation. The assembly is then dried in a preheated porcelain furnace (200°F) for 15 minutes (the door is left open to permit steam to escape).

After being completely dried, the invested units are pulled out onto the furnace platform for final examination, making sure the sluice ways are clear and porcelain is free of investment. At this time all surfaces of full-cast units to be soldered must be fluxed thoroughly. Porcelain veneer units need not be fluxed. The heat from the investment will melt and spread the flux evenly over the surface to be soldered. The units are then placed back into the preheated furnace and with the door partially opened, the temperature is raised to 1,250°F (50°/min). After heat soaking at 1,250°F for 2 minutes, the temperature is raised to 1,550°F (75°F/min).

While the temperature climbs, the soldering torch is activated (gas and air) and a thin strip of solder is covered with a thin layer of flux, which helps its flowability. The flame is brought to a very fine blue tip to maintain maximum heat. At 1,550°F, the invested case is pulled out onto the furnace platform or door with the labial and buccal porcelain surfaces facing and in close proximity to the inside of the furnace. The temperature on the inside of the furnace is permitted to rise in order to maintain a constant temperature on the porcelain surface. At this time, in most cases, the temperature of the investment and metal substructure is sufficient to melt the solder strip upon contact. However, to better control solder flow and to ensure that each contact is hot enough, the thin blue flame tip of the torch is directed to each connection immediately preceding the introduction of solder. The surfaces are heated and as the solder strip is fed to the connection, the flame is moved to the next one, taking care not to contact solder or porcelain. This can be done rapidly, completing an entire arch (15 connections) within 20 seconds.

Melted solder flows to the hottest spot; the added heat produced by the torch plus the heat from the furnace pulls the solder throughout the entire interproximal area. This method makes it possible to completely control solder flow in that while the torch and furnace supply the needed heat, the technician is able to regulate the amount of solder for each connection and also its direction of flow. The technician is able to watch as the

solder flows and can make absolutely certain that the connection is dense and free from porosity.

A postfabrication soldered restoration with a noble metal alloy substructure is strong enough to carry any load developed by normal occlusion and function and is highly recommended for cases that would be otherwise impossible to obtain individuality.

Cost Differential

Economy should not take priority over the patient's oral health; when comparing noble with base metal alloy, however, there is certainly a great price difference. Even though the price of most noble metal alloys exceeds that of base metal alloys by three or four times, the decision to use either should not be made because of price alone. Each case must be evaluated for its needs such as strength, hardness, tissue and wear factors, and whether or not postsoldering will be involved. Only on these requirements should the choice be made.

Nickel and Beryllium

Most base metal alloys used today contain nickel and beryllium. Although they are important ingredients, their toxicity is questioned. Some feel that nickel is harmful to the patient and beryllium to the technician. It is indeed true that some patients are allergic to nickel, but it is felt by many in the dental profession that there are not enough allergic patients to warrant banning its use. Also, although beryllium is considered a potential danger to the technician's health, proponents claim there are many other contaminants in the laboratory and if not properly eliminated from the work area, their effects can be just as harmful.

Regardless whether these two elements warrant concern, noble metal alloy is an alternative to base metal alloy, and if the dentist voices a concern, this alone should be the determining factor and reason enough to use noble metal alloys exclusively.

After having used base metal alloys for many years, I have experienced virtually no negative results due to the presence of nickel and beryllium. A simple nickel sensitivity test can be made on patients who show signs of allergy, while the laboratory can exert extra effort to eliminate grindings and dust left during metal finishing.

Summary

When function of a restoration is discussed, the metal substructure is seldom mentioned. In fact, the substructure is the basic foundation for function. A faulty metal substructure could cause a restoration to fail regardless of how much effort is placed on other aspects of the restoration.

Alloy selection and metal substructure design are therefore of prime importance and should not be taken lightly.

In comparing noble with base metal alloys, advantages and disadvantages are found in each. Quality control, hardness, strength, tissue and wear, veneer advantage, pre- and postfabrication soldered connections, economy, and the inclusion of nickel and beryllium should be recognized. In order to make the best alloy selection, all of the above attributes must be explored. This, coupled with a well-engineered metal substructure, will ensure success for any restoration.

Chapter 3

Composite Tooth Color

Dentistry today, more than ever, focuses greatly on function and esthetics. The last 60 years have brought about many advances in equipment, techniques, and materials (Figs 3-1a to c). Casting a gold crown by hand slinging melted alloy versus the same procedure using automatic induction and vacuum-pressure-type casting machines, and firing porcelain in a simple kiln versus using the highly sophisticated computerized, programmable furnaces of today, are just two examples of how dental technology has progressed. Many new alloys have been made available for the dentist and technician to choose from; improved investments have made precise castings more predictable; and porcelains have shown marked changes in strength, translucency, and consistency. Advancements in bonding and composite resins, along with new materials, have increased the possibility of improving esthetics tremendously. Removable partial dentures have progressed from being simple clasp types to embracing more esthetic and reliable precision attachment designs that can accommodate the most complicated case.

Yet despite the many changes and improvements that have taken place in dentistry regarding function and esthetics, tooth color analysis and duplication have remained untouched by similar change and improvement. Tooth color may not be considered as important as tooth contour when evaluating esthetics; however, color can make the difference between a mediocre restoration and an ultimately esthetic restoration. Unfortunately, there has been practically no change in concept or technique in analyzing and duplicating tooth color. Little effort has been made to determine the physiological components of tooth color, how the eye perceives these components, and how they can be translated into the language of ceramics. Even less has been accomplished in how to convey this information from the dentist to the laboratory.

Since the 1930s, the dental profession has based its entire concept of color on the "commercial shade guide." Shade guides are designed to serve as an aid in selecting denture teeth for removable full and partial dentures. Each tab—which is a sample of a denture tooth that is available in that particular shade—is made up of layers of porcelain that vary in color and location. Some of the problems found with shade guides are:

1. The porcelain and color oxides that form the tab are high-fusing (approximately 2,400°F) and are the same materials found in denture teeth. These materials in no way resemble the much lower-fusing porcelains (approximately 1,785°F) that are used for ceramic restorations.
2. Many shade tabs are coated with a surface stain in the gingival area and are mounted to a metal handle.
3. The effect from the opaque and metal backing, which make up part of the 1.5-mm-thick porcelain veneer, is not represented in the shade tab.
4. Shade guides from the same manufacturer vary from guide to guide and seldom corre-

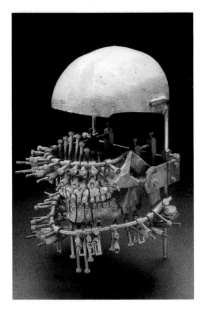

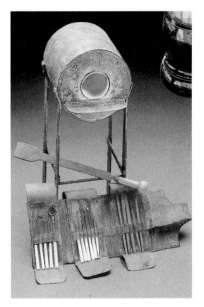

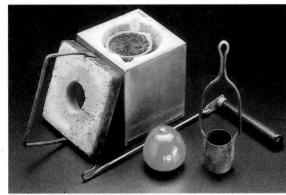

Fig 3-1a

Fig 3-1b

Fig 3-1c

Fig 3-1a One of the earliest instruments used for articulating models of the maxilla and mandible; it was used to study the relationship between the gliding surfaces of the teeth and jaw articulations and was adjustable in any spatial direction. There have been many changes and improvements made since the early 1900s, from this to the sophisticated, fully adjustable articulators of today. (Courtesy of Wolfgang O. Funk.)

Fig 3-1b Porcelain kiln used in 1910 to fire porcelain teeth. The kiln was heated with gas from below and behind, and although efficient, it is no match for the modern, computerized, automatic porcelain furnaces that can be preset for 100 different programs. The newer, improved furnaces are accurate to a fraction of a degree and are responsible for producing high-quality ceramic restorations. (Courtesy of Wolfgang O. Funk.)

Fig 3-1c Casting system used in the early 1900s. The furnace had a metal housing with a fire clay lining and was heated with a gas flame through a hole in the metal housing. The gold was melted in the crucible and centrifuged by hand, forcing the molten gold into the hollow mold after the wax pattern was burned out. There is quite a contrast between this and the induction casting systems of today. (Courtesy of Wolfgang O. Funk.)

spond exactly with the denture teeth they are supposed to match.

5. The average shade guide has a selection of 12 to 15 tabs to choose from, and even if a tab should be found that closely resembles the color of the tooth, the possibility of duplicating it exactly is remote; it is impossible to transfer all the color information found on a 5-mm-thick color tab to a 1-mm-thick restoration.

Because of these reasons, an entirely different approach to color must be initiated.

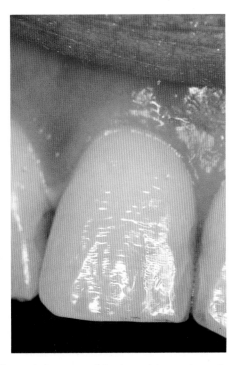

Fig 3-2a Maxillary right central incisor. Natural tooth color appears to be on the surface of the tooth or within its enamel. Actually, dentin is the source of tooth color; enamel is colorless. Colors in the dentin combine and project through the enamel. These combined colors become the composite tooth color (CTC).

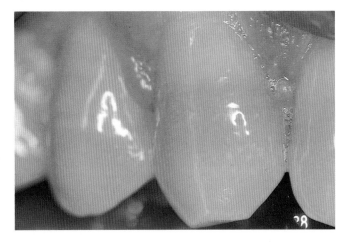

Fig 3-2b Maxillary right canine and premolar displaying a concentrated CTC. Tooth color differs from mouth to mouth, depends on the age and condition of the dentin, and varies from bland, almost colorless to dark and pronounced. In this example the effects of tetracycline are obvious and greatly influence the CTC.

Composite Tooth Color

A logical beginning to solving the tooth color problem would be to learn and understand what comprises tooth color and where color is located. "Composite tooth color" (CTC) can be defined as that color or colors located beneath the enamel and projected through it (Figs 3-2a and b). The following facts must be noted:

1. Two direct factors responsible for CTC are dentin and enamel. *Dentin* forms the bulk of the tooth. *Enamel* is colorless and although it does not contribute color to CTC, it regulates its value.

2. CTC is made up of color or colors located beneath the enamel layer, the main or basic color being that of the dentin. The dentin, therefore, is the predominant influence on CTC. If this was the only source of color, CTC duplication would be simple. However, there are other colors located in the dentin of most teeth that add to the complexity of CTC. I refer to these colors as *maverick colors* and define them as color or colors found in the dentin but not directly responsible for the dentin color; they combine with basic dentin color and project their resultant effect through the enamel as CTC. They also appear in different areas of the dentin, representing certain color families in several degrees of concentration but with no set rule or pattern. The family colors are narrow in spectrum (yellow, honey yellow, light, and dark brown)

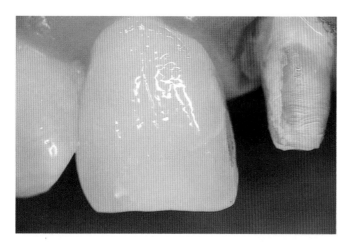

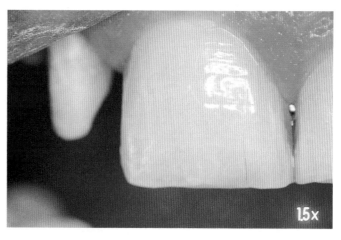

Fig 3-3a Prepared maxillary left central incisor as compared to the unprepared right central incisor. The CTC of the right central incisor is the result of the combined dentin and maverick colors. The embedded light brown maverick color is obvious and influences the CTC even though dentin is the main contributor.

Fig 3-3b Prepared maxillary right central incisor compared to unprepared left central incisor. The maverick colors are less concentrated than those in Fig 3-3a but are just as important a component of CTC. Maverick concentration varies from subtle to highly concentrated but is usually limited to the same color family found throughout the dental arch.

but vary in concentration. The influence that maverick colors exert on CTC ranges from subtle to extensive, depending on their saturation (Figs 3-3a and b).

3. Enamel acts as a transmitter of the underlying color found in the dentin and is made up of long rods that are surrounded by a prismatic substance and are perpendicular to the dentin. It is through the combined efforts of these rods and interprismatic substance that a fiberoptic type system exists that is able to reflect, absorb, and transmit light. This fiberoptic arrangement permits light to pass through the enamel, strike the underlying color found at the dentinoenamel junction, and reflect it in all directions. The color or colors perceived as such can be referred to as CTC. As previously mentioned, enamel is colorless. Any degree of color observed on the surface or within the confines of the enamel should be classified as an irregularity, and although it cannot be regarded as a component of CTC, it must be incorporated in the restoration (Figs 3-4 and 3-5).

4. Some teeth, especially those found in younger patients, have little or no maverick influence (Fig 3-6).

5. In general, dentin and maverick colors vary only in saturation throughout the mouth. The difference in color concentration is caused mainly by the difference in thickness from tooth to tooth. Canines, because they are bulky, are usually the "darkest" teeth in the mouth; mandibular incisors, which are less bulky, are the "lightest." Posterior teeth may be bulkier than canines, but the abundance of enamel contained in posterior teeth tends to diminish much of the color influence found beneath it. It is important to note, however, that although color concentrations vary from tooth to tooth in any given mouth, color families tend to be the same and any change during duplication will be recognized immediately (Figs 3-7 and 3-8).

6. The color spectrum of dentin varies mainly in saturation. Color intensity will increase with age but the color family will not change.

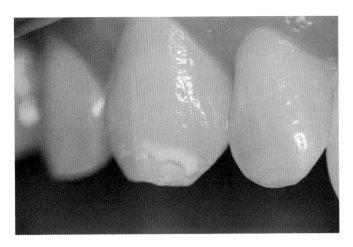

Fig 3-4 Maxillary right canine and lateral incisor with different degrees of hypocalcification in the enamel of the incisal third of each. The canine contains a more concentrated area of this irregularity than the lateral incisor. This is one of several irregularities commonly found in the enamel layer and is not considered a component of CTC.

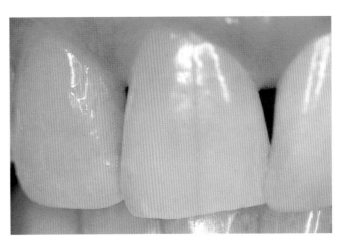

Fig 3-5 Maxillary right central and lateral incisors with enamel irregularities. Lateral incisor: subtle hypocalcification, several craze lines, and mesial interproximal discoloration. Central incisor: hypocalcification and light brown check line. Any irregularity found in the enamel, although not responsible for CTC, must be included in the restoration in order for it to harmonize with the remaining natural dentition.

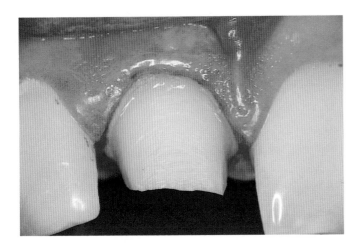

Fig 3-6 Prepared maxillary right central incisor of a young patient. Close observation shows dentin with no visible maverick colors. In cases such as this where maverick colors are absent, only three color dimensions are involved in the CTC: hue, chroma, and value.

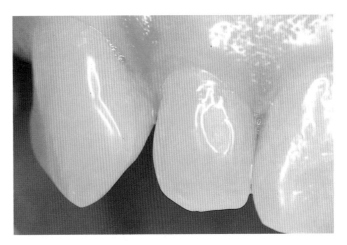

Fig 3-7 Color concentration of maxillary right canine compared to the lateral incisor. The same family color is obvious in both teeth, as is the difference in concentration. It is logical to assume that the bulkier canine, with more dentin thickness, will display more concentrated color than thinner teeth throughout the mouth.

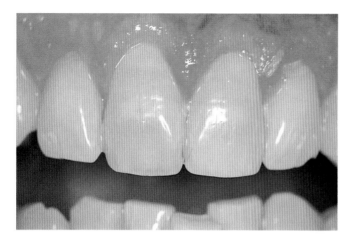

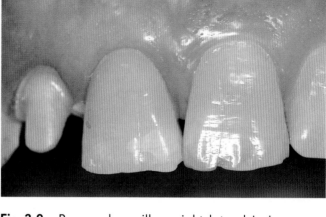

Fig 3-8 Maxillary four incisors with a common CTC but variety in color concentration. Note obvious difference between the central incisors. Although the family color persists in the four incisors, four different degrees of saturation exist. Therefore, when duplicating a natural dentition, it is more important to establish the exact color family and less important to duplicate exact color concentration. In fact, a full-arch restoration having a uniform color concentration is less realistic.

Fig 3-9 Prepared maxillary right lateral incisor compared to the unprepared central incisors, the only difference being the influence enamel has on CTC. If we can accept a broad definition of hue as basic color, hue can be assigned to the dentin of the tooth. Note how the dentin color is projected through the enamel of the unprepared central incisors. Once the dentin color (hue) has been established, any diluted version can be referred to as the chroma.

The Four Dimensional Tooth Color System

In order to duplicate CTC, the colors responsible for creating the CTC must be recognizable and a system must be devised to convey the information to the laboratory. A logical approach would be to treat tooth color much like an artist treats color. Artists describe color in terms of dimension: hue, chroma and value (much like a carpenter recognizes length, height, and depth). These dimensions are discussed as follows.

Hue—The First Color Dimension

Broadly, hue is the basic color of an object. Because dentin makes up the bulk of the tooth, it is reasonable to say that it is most responsible for CTC. Further, the color contributed by the dentin can be considered the basic color of that tooth. Therefore, the dimension *hue* can be assigned to the *dentin* of the tooth. This establishes the first dimension and the color most responsible for CTC. As you look at an unprepared tooth, the predominant color can occasionally be recognized and defined as dentin color or hue, but as will be described later, could be confused with other colors in the dentin (maverick colors) that combine with the hue to form CTC (Fig 3-9). (Readers should also refer to: Muia PJ. *The Four Dimensional Tooth Color System*. Chicago, Quintessence Publ Co, 1982.)

Chroma—The Second Color Dimension

Chroma is defined as a further refinement of hue. Chroma is a desaturated or diluted version of hue that automatically associates it with the dentin. It becomes the second color dimension and signifies the strength of hue while maintaining basic color. This close relationship between the hue and chroma dimensions permits combining them into what could be called *hue-chroma*. This makes it possible to dilute a hue that is found to be too concentrated when describing the dentin. For example, if the dentin is classified as a specific hue (basic color) but not quite as intense, the chroma version of that particular hue can be designated as its hue-chroma dimension, and it is this dimension that becomes the dominant factor in the CTC of that tooth.

Maverick—The Third Color Dimension

As already mentioned, all the colors beneath the enamel make up CTC. Although the dentin (hue-chroma dimension) is the most influential, the *maverick* colors contribute tremendously to it; so much so that ignorance of this dimension could make the difference between success and failure in CTC duplication. The maverick colors that are most important are those located at the dentinoenamel junction. These colors combine with the dentin and produce the CTC. Maverick colors located deeper into the dentin have little effect on CTC. The relatively narrow color range found in natural dentition makes it easy to recognize and duplicate maverick colors (see Figs 3-3a and b).

Value—The Fourth Color Dimension

The entire crown of the tooth is covered with enamel. Enamel itself is colorless, but through its network of rods it projects the underlying color found in the dentin. Value is defined as brightness and theoretically ranges from white (high value) to black (low value). *Value* is assigned to enamel because enamel covers the underlying tooth, modifying its brightness. Enamel is thus the fourth color dimension responsible for CTC.

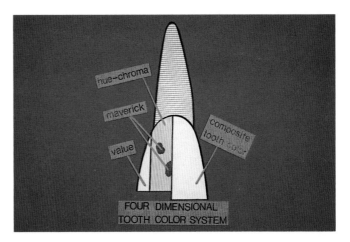

Fig 3-10 The four color dimensions can be found in all vital dentitions. In order to accurately duplicate CTC, a method for detecting and measuring these color dimensions is essential. By removing at least part of the enamel down to the dentin enamel junction, access will be obtained to these color dimensions and the observer will be able to make a more reliable evaluation.

The Four Dimensional Tooth Color System thus takes advantage of the dimensions of color. Hue, which designates the basic family color, is further refined to its chroma through desaturation, combines with the maverick dimension, and passes through the enamel, which regulates its value, to materialize as CTC. A prime objective in a ceramic restoration is to duplicate CTC. Reproducing the four color dimensions exactly as found in the tooth will assure a near-perfect duplication of CTC. In order to accomplish this, these dimensions must be recognized (detected) and evaluated (measured).

Detecting the Color Dimensions

Detection of the hue-chroma and maverick dimensions requires at least partial removal of the enamel to the dentinoenamel junction (Fig 3-10). The enamel obscures the underlying color and

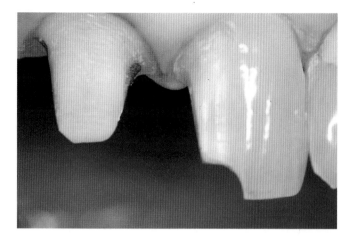

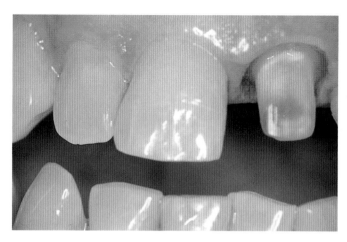

Fig 3-11 Fully prepared maxillary right incisor and semiprepared left central incisor. The semiprepared left central incisor shows the effect enamel has on CTC. It also aids when deciding which duplicating method will be best. Note same color family in both central incisors. Exposed dentin, whether it be fully prepared or semiprepared tooth, is necessary for accurate color detection.

Fig 3-12 Prepared maxillary left central incisor. Hue, chroma, and maverick color dimensions are easily detected when the maverick dimension is this pronounced (light brown at the middle third). The basic color family (hue-chroma) can be seen in the remaining dentin color. It would be impossible to detect these color dimensions using the unprepared right central incisor as a source. The enamel has distributed the spot of maverick color uniformly throughout the entire tooth. This must be taken into consideration when selecting the appropriate duplicating method.

makes it difficult to accurately detect the hue-chroma and maverick dimensions. When possible, it is advisable to retain part of the enamel in the form of a partial covering. This permits comparison between the prepared section with the unprepared section, showing what influence the enamel has on CTC. Also, it presents an opportunity to measure the value dimension (Fig 3-11).

Color detection must be accurate, as must be its measurement in order for it to be precisely duplicated.

Detecting Hue

In detecting the hue, it is important to distinguish the dentin color from the maverick color. Even though the maverick color may be more intense or

outstanding, the dentin color (hue) transmits the family color. Beneath the enamel layer, these dimensions are separate and must be treated as such. In terms of CTC, however, they are observed differently; they combine their efforts and project their resultant effect through the enamel. The enamel, being a translucent covering, will not alter the basic hue or color family of the maverick; it regulates the value or brightness while its blanket-like quality tends to soften or muffle the underlying color, thus making it somewhat more difficult to recognize the color dimensions (Fig 3-12).

The rather narrow spectrum of color found in normal healthy dentin falls into two general categories: (1) yellow-orange and (2) orange-brown. These vary only in saturation (strength). Even teeth that appear to be in the so called "gray family" contain some concentration of yellow, orange, or brown. Grayness is attributed to value (brightness) and should not be evaluated as hue. The presence of these colors ranges from a very low concentration, where the color is almost impossible to identify, to such a high concentration that the color must be classified as maverick. The dentin in most young teeth is low in color concentration. Age and physiological change tend to increase color concentration. Other contributing factors include diet, medication, heredity, and enamel wear. Of these, enamel wear, whether brought about normally or by malocclusion, will show the most rapid rate of increased color concentration. Once the protective enamel layer is worn to the point of dentin exposure, especially at the incisal edges of anterior teeth, the relatively soft spongy dentin absorbs color from foods, beverages, and mouth fluids. Color accumulates first at the worn incisal edges and gradually works its way through the porous dentin until the entire tooth exhibits color change. These colors, without exception, are found to be in the orange and brown color range and vary considerably in saturation. In most cases of enamel wear, the hue will change more rapidly than in teeth that retain enamel protection.

Although the removal of part of the enamel helps in detecting hue, in some cases color dimension detection can be accomplished very well in unprepared teeth. This is especially true in teeth with high color concentration that involve just two dimensions, maverick and value (Figs 3-13a to c).

After detecting the hue dimension and placing it into its proper color family (yellow, orange, or brown), the next step is to determine the chroma (degree of saturation).

Detecting Chroma

Upon detecting the hue, further refinement might be necessary. If the hue dimension is considered to be the most saturated version of a particular color, any version less concentrated would be referred to as chroma. If an accurate hue selection is made and no further effort is made to refine it, the finished selection will, without a doubt, be acceptable. In general, the hue remains the same throughout the mouth, while the chroma may vary greatly. Chroma determination simply ensures a more accurate CTC duplication. For this reason, the two dimensions are combined to be referred to as hue-chroma (see Figs 3-7 and 3-8).

Detecting Maverick

Most teeth will have the third color dimension, maverick. Maverick colors are easily detected and may vary in concentration from tooth to tooth. Colors such as green, blue, pink, and red are seldom if ever found in the dentin. When these colors are used in a ceramic restoration they contribute nothing to the naturalness of the restoration. Only the maverick colors at the dentino-enamel junction are contributors to CTC. Without the enamel covering, the hue-chroma and maverick dimensions are detected as separate entities and are easily recognized as such. The enamel covering, with its fiberoptic capabilities, combines these colors and in most cases makes it difficult to recognize them individually. Maverick colors can be referred to as variables in respect to CTC in that they vary the effects of the hue-chroma dimension; hue-chroma projected through enamel would differ only in value or brightness when comparing dentin color to composite tooth color. Maverick influence, however, could alter the dentin influence on CTC greatly. Its effect could range from subtle to very obvious. For this reason, the maverick dimension could, in many cases, be considered more influential to CTC than the hue-chroma dimension (see Fig 3-12).

Partial removal of the enamel makes maverick detection simple, the most important factor being selecting the correct color family and concentration.

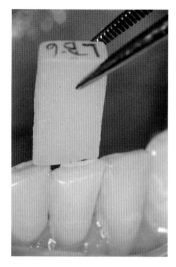

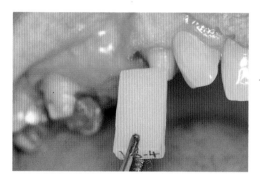

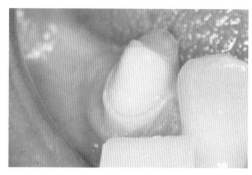

Fig 3-13a   **Fig 3-13b**   **Fig 3-13c**

Fig 3-13a Mandibular anterior teeth with worn enamel at the incisal edge and exposed dentin. Once the dentin has been exposed, discoloration of the dentin is relatively rapid, beginning at the incisal edge and eventually engulfing the entire dentin. Enamel erosion at the gingival third of the tooth will bring about the same results. Note the maverick color tab and how well it compares to the underlying dentin. In this case, just two dimensions are detected: maverick and value.

Fig 3-13b Prepared maxillary right first premolar exposing dentin that was found to be in the maverick color range. As the dentin discolored, the hue-chroma dimension gradually disappeared and eventually gave way to the maverick dimension. The restoration will consist of two dimensions: maverick (dentin) and value (enamel). Note how well the maverick color tab matches both the prepared premolar and the unprepared canine.

Fig 3-13c Prepared mandibular right premolar with maverick color tab (maverick and value dimensions). When restoring a full arch, a diluted version of the detected maverick color can produce excellent esthetic results. The neutral porcelain needed to de-saturate the maverick selection and the full enamel coverage permits more light to enter deep into the restoration and render it vibrant and lifelike.

Detecting Value

The effect the enamel has on CTC becomes evident when you compare the prepared half to the unprepared half of a tooth. The dentinoenamel junction displays the individual color components (hue-chroma and maverick dimensions) that combine to manifest as CTC. The semiprepared tooth gives immediate access to this information and makes detection straightforward and uncomplicated. The colorless enamel has no direct effect on these color dimensions but does indirectly affect CTC by its ability to combine their efforts and project their results.

It must be remembered that normal enamel is colorless; any color found in the enamel, during detection, is there because of an irregularity that was brought about either during tooth development or after eruption. When attempting to duplicate exactly what is found during detection, these irregularities must be included in the restoration.

Measuring the Color Dimensions

Once the four color dimensions have been detected they must be measured. In order to duplicate the color dimensions, a standard gauge or measuring device must be established so that the information can be accurately conveyed to the laboratory. The prepared teeth should be kept in a wet state while measuring the color dimensions.

The CTC Guide as a Measuring "Device"

The inadequacy of the commercial shade guide makes it imperative that a more reliable means for measuring tooth color dimension be established. This is accomplished with a customized tooth color guide. The customized guide is an organized collection of porcelain samples made up of tabs that display the materials that can be made available by the laboratory and that match the four tooth color dimensions. Four separate guides, one corresponding to each of the four tooth color dimensions, should be constructed with the porcelains that will be used for the restoration. Each tab is a sample of what the ceramist is capable of producing with a given porcelain and technique. If the dentist is able to match a particular tab with that color dimension found in the tooth, it is reasonable to assume that the ceramist can duplicate it in the restoration.

The CTC guide can be patterned after any commercial shade guide using the same nomenclature, which must correspond to the porcelain used in the laboratory. However, there are some distinct differences between the CTC guide and a commercial shade guide:

1. The CTC guide is a more realistic approach to measuring tooth color dimension because the porcelains used to construct it are the same porcelains used in the restoration. This is not the case with commercial shade guides, which are made from high-fusing porcelains used primarily for constructing denture teeth.
2. The CTC guide measures individual color dimensions separately; the commercial shade guide, on the other hand, attempts to clump them all together with no concern for color concentration or location.
3. The thickness of the customized color tab is the same as that of the restoration (1.5 mm). The commercial tab measures as much as 4 to 5 mm.

The customized tooth color guide, therefore, acts as a standard measuring "device" that incorporates all the tangible and intangible ingredients necessary to quantify the four tooth color dimensions. It acts as a communicating aid to be used between the dentist and laboratory. The dentist is able to describe in detail exactly what is needed to duplicate CTC.

Measuring Hue

Because dentin is the strongest contributor to composite tooth color, it is the most logical dimension to measure first. Dentin supplies the family color, therefore the customized tab that is used to measure this dimension must be one that consists of porcelain made up of family dentin color. Every porcelain kit contains dentin porcelain that is bottled according to color and patterned after a particular commercial shade guide (eg, B65, A3, P3). The customized tab is made by firing body porcelain (dentin) over its prescribed opaque and is taken directly out of the bottle with no modification. The tab represents exactly what can be expected in the final restoration. When the dentist is able to match it perfectly with the dentin of the tooth, the ceramist is certain it can be duplicated.

It is important to accurately measure the hue dimension so that it establishes the correct family color (usually either yellow, orange, or brown). Should the selection be inaccurate, the CTC could be greatly affected.

If during the detection stage you find that the dentin color does not fall into any of the hue ranges due to high concentration of color, it will be necessary to rely on the maverick guide, which is made up of color modifiers and will be discussed later. If the hue tab is the proper family but the color is too concentrated, the chroma guide must come into play.

Measuring Chroma

Chroma, as a further refinement of hue, is used only when the hue selection is found to be too concentrated. The chroma customized tab is made by adding one portion of neutral porcelain to several portions of dentin porcelain, using opaque at full strength. Along with desaturating the hue, the neutral porcelain separates the color particles, permitting more light to enter into the crown, thus encouraging more light diffusion and a more lifelike restoration. Each hue is desaturated by adding one part of neutral porcelain to three parts of body (dentin) porcelain. This gives the dentist a choice of four degrees of saturation of any given hue: (1) fully saturated tab, (2) three parts of dentin porcelain to one part neutral tab, (3) a desaturated version between the fully saturated tab and the three to one tab (four to one), and (4) a very desaturated version (two to one).

Thus, a fully saturated hue tab and one chroma tab (three to one), makes it possible to choose from four versions of each hue.

When finding that the basic hue is too concentrated when compared to the dentin, the chroma tab (three parts of dentin porcelain to one part neutral) is engaged. If this tab is found to be overdiluted, the selection will automatically fall between it and the fully saturated hue (four parts dentin to one part neutral). If it is too concentrated, the logical selection would be the more desaturated version (two parts dentin porcelain to one part neutral).

When it is necessary to select a desaturated version of the hue (chroma), the hue tab is no longer needed and the chroma tab will dictate the body buildup (dentin porcelain) of the restoration, regardless which duplication method is used. The chroma tab now represents the hue-chroma dimension and tells the ceramist how many parts of dentin porcelain should be added to one part of neutral porcelain, while also pointing out the prescribed opaque for that particular hue to be used as the first opaque wash (Fig 3-14).

Once the hue-chroma dimension has been measured, the next step is to search out any maverick color that might be present.

Measuring Maverick

If no maverick is present in the dentin, duplicating the CTC is uncomplicated because it depends on only two dimensions: hue (or chroma) and value. However, when maverick colors are detected, duplicating the CTC becomes more complicated because the hue-chroma and maverick dimensions combine their efforts with the value dimension (enamel) to form CTC.

The maverick shade guide is constructed with body modifiers and neutral porcelain. This differs from the hue and chroma guides in that opaque is not used. Modifiers from any porcelain kit can be used, and only four color families are necessary: yellow, orange, light brown, and dark brown (Fig 3-15). These are the only maverick colors found in teeth; the other modifiers such as green, blue, and red are useless and could cause confusion when attempting to measure the four tooth color dimensions.

The first tab of each of the four maverick colors is made to full saturation, that is, with no neutral

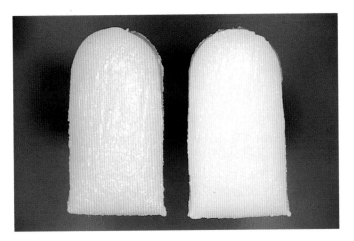

Fig 3-14 Hue *(left)* and chroma *(right)* tabs of a tooth color family. The first step in measuring the four tooth color dimensions is to find the dentin color family. The matching customized hue tab denotes the basic color family but not necessarily its exact concentration. When the hue measurement needs further refinement, the chroma tab (a desaturated version of the hue) is used to determine the portions of dentin and neutral porcelain that must be used in the restoration to produce a perfect duplication of the CTC.

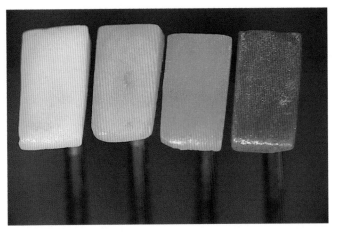

Fig 3-15 Four fully saturated customized maverick color tabs. Each tab represents a color family (yellow, orange, light brown, and dark brown) derived from the body modifiers of the porcelain system. Maverick colors are seldom found in dentin in a fully saturated state; they are usually found in a diluted form, even when the entire dentin has darkened to the maverick dimension range (customized maverick color tabs have no opaque layer).

porcelain added. This tab will represent the color family of that particular maverick and will determine the maverick color family found in the tooth. The body modifier is taken from the bottle and mixed with the liquid prescribed by the manufacturer. It should be condensed using the same method used routinely during porcelain buildup. This is transferred to the Williams Shade Tab Former (Williams Gold Co) and condensed further, blotting liquid until the tab can be removed and placed on a firing tray (covered with a sagger tray liner). The firing temperature should be slightly below the maturing temperature of the body modifier. The same procedure is used for the remaining three modifiers.

The first desaturated tab is made up of one part body modifier mixed with one part neutral porcelain. This tab represents a 50% dilution of the original tab and marks the beginning of a shade guide that is progressively desaturated from tab to tab.

The next tab is made up of one part body modifier to two parts neutral porcelain. Each tab is diluted with an added part of neutral porcelain and should be taken to seven dilutions (one part of body modifier to seven parts neutral porcelain) (Fig 3-16). This makes a total of eight tabs for each maverick color family and a full maverick shade guide consisting of 32 tabs.

The maverick shade guide is just as critical as the hue and chroma guide and in many cases is more critical when measuring and duplicating CTC. It also serves as a sole measuring device when the dentin color is found to be completely out of the range of the hue or chroma guide and only maverick and value are responsible for the CTC. With its unlimited possible combinations, the maverick shade guide can help you select colors

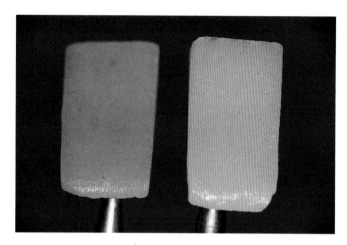

Fig 3-16 Two light brown maverick shade tabs. The tab on the left is LB, fully saturated; the tab on the right is LB-3, made up of one part light brown and three parts neutral porcelain. Note the degree of desaturation when neutral porcelain is added. As many as eight parts of neutral porcelain can be added to one part of body modifier to achieve needed color.

for full maxillary or mandibular arch restorations where body buildup (dentin) is accomplished entirely with body modifiers covered over with enamel porcelain.

The entire maverick shade guide, from the fully saturated tab, which is used to measure high concentrations of maverick colors, to the most desaturated tab used to measure subtle areas of color, is an integral tool for measuring and duplicating CTC. Without it, communicating true tooth color is impossible.

The first step in measuring the maverick dimension is to determine the family color (yellow, orange, light brown, or dark brown) by comparing it to a fully saturated maverick tab. This is important because an accurate initial selection will determine the color dominance which, when combined with the hue-chroma, places the CTC into a particular color family. Even though the dentin is the bulkiest part of the tooth and is the prime contributor to the CTC, the incorporation of maverick color makes the difference between a

mediocre restoration and one that exhibits perfect CTC duplication.

The second step is to measure the exact dilution of the family maverick selection. If the initial selected tab is of satisfactory concentration (fully saturated), there is no need to go further. If the fully saturated tab is too concentrated, however, (which is usually the case), tabs that are progressively less saturated should be tried until the tab matching the maverick color concentration is found. This should be recorded, along with the hue-chroma tab selection, noting the parts of neutral porcelain that were mixed with one part of modifier to construct this tab.

It is important to note exactly how the detected maverick influences the CTC. This can be accomplished by comparing the prepared half of the tooth with the unprepared half. The prepared half reveals the exact family, concentration, and location, while the unprepared half shows the effect of the enamel covering and how the maverick color has combined with hue-chroma to form the CTC. This presents the ceramist with information required for determining the appropriate duplicating method. For example, one spot of maverick color located beneath the enamel could influence the entire CTC uniformly or it could influence it only in the immediate area. The fiberoptic-like effect of the enamel makes it possible for the enamel to pick up a spot of maverick color and display its effects uniformly throughout the entire tooth. Maverick color often affects CTC by exhibiting areas of color concentration rather than influencing it uniformly. The effect maverick has on CTC dictates the method that will best duplicate CTC.

The selected maverick tab represents the third measured dimension. The fourth and last dimension to be measured is value.

Measuring Value

Comparing the prepared half of the tooth with the unprepared half will show how the enamel influences the CTC. Under normal conditions, enamel is colorless; thus its only contribution to CTC is brightness or lack of it.

The value shade guide is made up of tabs of enamel porcelain with measured parts of gray modifier. A measuring device with two capacities is necessary (approximately 10 to 1). The first tab consists of enamel porcelain with the highest value (no gray added). The second tab is made up of one large part of enamel porcelain and one small part of gray (1/10 of the enamel portion). The third tab is made of one large part enamel porcelain to two small parts gray. As the number of value tabs increase, an additional small portion of gray is mixed with one large portion of enamel porcelain. Each successive shade tab decreases in value as more gray is added. The value shade guide should be carried to at least four tabs with several additional tabs of quite low value that must accommodate restorations to be placed next to teeth with amalgam fillings.

The enamel regulates the value of the CTC as the hue-chroma dimensions are projected through it. The enamel of most teeth is of high value and can therefore be measured quite accurately using the higher end of the shade guide. The lower end of the value guide is seldom used for this reason but is necessary for abnormalities and for blending purposes (with adjacent teeth).

Value should be measured during the semi-preparation stage or at some other convenient time when a section of enamel is exposed behind which there is no dentin. To accurately measure value, the enamel must be free of color influence or any other condition that could distort the true brightness of the tooth. The location that best accomplishes this is the extreme mesial or distal area of the tooth. Occasionally, the incisal edge can be used after the dentin has been removed in this area, using the lingual enamel surface. The value tab that matches the brightness of the enamel designates how many small parts of gray body modifier must be added to one large part of enamel porcelain to exactly duplicate the brightness of the tooth.

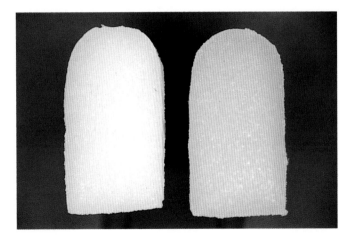

Fig 3-17 Two customized value tabs show contrast between high and low value. The tab on the left is fabricated with the enamel porcelain of highest value in the porcelain system. The tab on the right has small parts of gray added to lower the value. When tabs of higher value are needed, parts of white body modifier are added (value tabs have no opaque layer).

Occasionally you may need a tab that is higher in value than the enamel porcelains supplied by the manufacturer. Some tooth enamel is extremely high in value, and in order to accurately measure it, value tabs made up of enamel porcelain and parts of white body modifier must be used.

The value tab selection is the final measurement and indicates the exact enamel porcelain formula needed to duplicate tooth brightness in the restoration (Fig 3-17).

Duplicating CTC

Once the more complicated procedures of detecting and measuring the four tooth color dimensions are completed, duplicating the CTC becomes rather routine and uncomplicated. It simply involves reproducing the three selected customized tooth color tabs (hue-chroma, maverick, and value) in the form of a ceramic restoration.

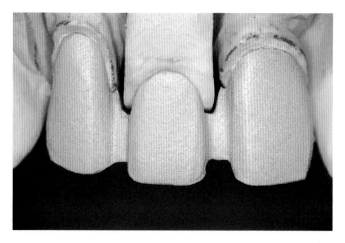

Fig 3-18 Maxillary three-unit restoration after the application of opaque has been fired. This opaque layer should be a thin, uniform covering that blocks out at least 50% of the underlying metal color. A slightly thicker layer may be necessary for alloys that develop a darker oxidation layer, as in the case of some base metal alloys.

There are eight methods for duplicating CTC. These methods will be repeated throughout the book, incorporating specific irregularities and techniques required to satisfy certain cases. Circumstances surrounding each case will determine the duplicating method best suited for it. Family color, concentration, location, and veneer thickness will help you to decide the most appropriate method for each case. The semiprepared tooth (half of the enamel removed from the labial/buccal surface to the dentinoenamel junction) will reveal the four tooth color dimensions. Comparing the prepared half with the unprepared half will show the effect the enamel has on the underlying color, thus helping to determine which duplicating method should be used. The unprepared half indicates how the color is displayed through the efforts of the enamel with its ability to transmit color in many directions.

Opaque

Success in duplicating CTC depends greatly on proper opaquing procedures. Many color failures in metal ceramic restorations can be attributed to the opaque layer. Opaque influences CTC so much that it could make the difference between a beautiful, lifelike restoration and one that is unacceptable. Opaque must not only contain the color dimensions that are necessary to obtain CTC, but it must also transmit them in such a way as to enhance the colors placed in the dentin so that their efforts are combined and displayed by the enamel. In order for opaque to accurately contribute to CTC, it should be applied in two separate firings, each having specific functions.

Opaque Layer

The opaque layer is a thin "wash" made up of the opaque corresponding to the selected hue-chroma dimension of the CTC. For instance, if A3, or any desaturated version of A3, was selected as the hue-chroma dimension for the restoration, A3 opaque would be thinly applied over the metal substructure and fired to the prescribed maturing temperature. This layer should be applied uniformly, covering the entire veneer surface and fired to a satin-like glaze (Fig 3-18). It serves several purposes:

1. It acts as a degassing procedure. The thin layer permits gases in the metal to escape while sealing the surface pores (a thick opaque layer could trap these gases in the form of minute pockets or porosity that would eventually cause bubbling and porcelain fracture during subsequent firings).
2. It blocks out approximately 50% of the underlying metal color influence.
3. It establishes a base material upon which dentin porcelain can be fired. Dentin porcelain should never be fired directly to metal; otherwise, inferior bonding could result.
4. It forms the beginning of the CTC.

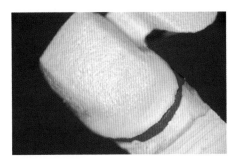

Fig 3-19a

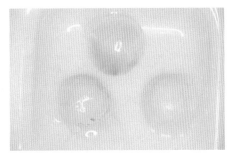

Fig 3-19b

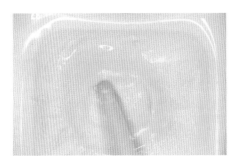

Fig 3-19c

Fig 3-19a Fired porcelain margin. When porcelain margins are involved in a restoration, it is necessary to fire the margin porcelain after the opaque layer is complete and before the transition of opaque is applied. Its maturing temperature is lower than that of the opaque wash and higher than that of the transition layer. Regardless which porcelain system is used, maturing temperatures should range from highest to lowest; that is, (1) opaque wash, (2) margin porcelain, (3) transition layer, and (4) body and enamel porcelain.

Fig 3-19b The ingredients for the transition layer are approximately one third each opaque, body porcelain, and modifier. The body modifier is the maverick selection made up of the proper portions of modifier and neutral porcelain. For instance, if the maverick dimension was LB-4 (one part light brown body modifier to four parts neutral porcelain), one third of the transition layer mixture would be made up of this.

Fig 3-19c Mixture for transition layer ready for application. Distilled water is used rather than buildup liquid because it is common to both body porcelain and opaque; buildup liquid could create a problem. The mixture should be thoroughly spatulated before application.

Transition Layer (Figs 3-19a to e)

The transition layer is the foundation upon which the CTC is built. It is made up of three components: opaque, dentin porcelain, and body modifier (maverick dimension). Because the opaque layer blocks out 50% of the metal color, only a small amount of opaque is needed to block out the remaining 50%. This affords an opportunity to begin building the four color dimensions into the transition layer of the restoration. Regardless which duplicating method is to be used, all color components should be included in the transition layer. The portions of each color component will vary, depending on the needs and restrictions associated with the restoration.

A general rule in proportioning the three ingredients that make up the transition layer is to use approximately one third each of opaque, dentin porcelain, and body modifier. If you need either more dentin (hue) or maverick influence, larger portions of each should be included. Of the three ingredients, opaque is usually used in smaller portions because the CTC is influenced more by hue than maverick, which requires a larger portion of dentin porcelain in the mixture. If the CTC needs to be influenced more by its maverick dimension, a larger portion of body modifier will be required. It is impossible to prescribe exact portions; much depends on the porcelain system used and the techniques used by the ceramist (eg, porcelain application, condensing, and firing). Expe-

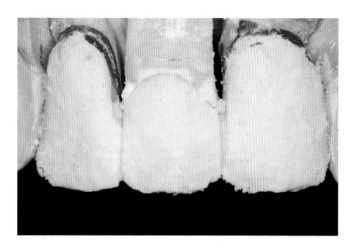

Fig 3-19d Transition layer before firing. While the transition layer is still in a semiwet state, a rough surface should be created, for instance with a stiff, short-bristle brush.

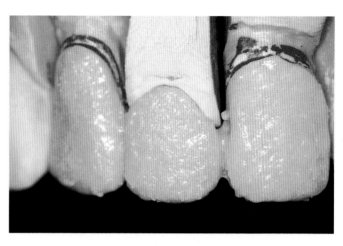

Fig 3-19e Fired transition layer. When fired at the proper temperature, the transition layer will maintain its rough surface, which is essential for diffusing light as it enters the restoration. Subsequent firings will not reach the maturing temperature of this layer, therefore the rough surface will remain and will not melt into the next firing.

rience and close observation will help when selecting exact portions for the transition layer.

There is one exception to the three ingredient rule, however. In many teeth the CTC is made up of only two color dimensions: maverick and value. In other words, the hue-chroma dimension is completely overpowered by the maverick dimension. In such cases, the dentin has darkened to the point where its hue-chroma dimension no longer falls into the hue range of the CTC guide; the maverick color guide must be used to measure this color dimension.

In cases such as this, the transition layer is composed of approximately one third opaque and two thirds body modifier (maverick dimension). The one third portion of opaque is sufficient to block out the remaining 50% of the metal color not covered by the opaque wash, white the two thirds portion of body modifier forms the foundation for the CTC.

The colors that are incorporated into the transition layer must be reflected in a diffused fashion.

This is accomplished by developing a rough surface during buildup. Light enters the restoration, penetrating the enamel and dentin porcelain, striking the rough surface, and reflects these colors back to the eye in a diffused fashion. This adds to the lifelike qualities of the restoration.

When adding body porcelain and modifiers to the transition layer, the maturing firing temperature must be lower than that of pure opaque. The difference should be between 10° and 15°, depending on the porcelain system used and the portions of each component (the larger the portions of body porcelain and modifiers, the lower the maturing temperature). It is important to not overfire the transition layer. Overfiring not only burns out needed colorants but also prohibits maximum masking of the metal substructure. When properly fired, the transition layer should resemble an "eggshell" finish.

After the transition layer is completed, the metal color should be eliminated and the CTC is practically accomplished. At this point, it should be difficult to recognize opacity; the transition layer should resemble dentin porcelain. The maturing temperature for the transition layer is higher than all subsequent firings; therefore, the roughened surface will retain its texture and will not "melt" during the dentin and enamel phase.

Eight Methods for Duplicating CTC

The eight methods for duplicating CTC are patterned after the maverick dimension. The choice of method for each restoration depends on the amount of influence the maverick dimension has on the CTC.

In the following exercise, six of these eight methods will be described in detail. The "no maverick technique" (#7) is used when the maverick dimension is not present. The "surface maverick technique" (#8) can be combined where needed with any of the other seven techniques. The purpose of the exercise is to show that although six different methods are used, the colors incorporated into the restorations can be quite harmonious. The methods vary, but the principles of the four tooth color dimensions remain the same.

The duplicating methods are distributed as follows:

Maxillary right central incisor:
    Maverick over opaque
Maxillary left lateral incisor #1:
    Embedded maverick
    Maverick plus hue-chroma
Maxillary left lateral incisor #2:
    Maverick buildup
    Maverick plus hue-chroma
Maxillary right canine #1:
    Deep stain maverick
Maxillary right canine #2:
    Maverick and enamel

Preparation for this exercise is shown in Figs 3-20a to c.

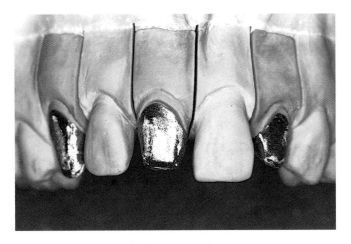

Fig 3-20a Dressed down castings, ready for final cleaning before porcelain application. Every successful restoration begins with a well-designed substructure. A full waxup with a sufficient cutback that ensures proper support for porcelain will help ensure a successful restoration. Needed thickness for a reliable substructure depends on the alloy used (precious metal, 0.3 mm; semiprecious metal, 0.2 mm; base metal [nonprecious], 0.1 mm).

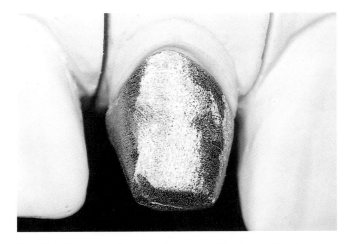

Fig 3-20b Maxillary right central incisor die showing proper preparation for a porcelain margin restoration. A 90-degree labial shoulder preparation is necessary when a porcelain margin is prescribed, regardless of which technique is used. To save time and material, the wax pattern should exclude the shoulder portion. When comparing the right and left central incisors, note the available room for porcelain application. All restorations in this exercise, including metal, opaque, transition layer, dentin, and enamel will measure less than 1 mm in thickness.

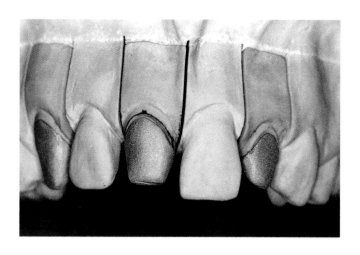

Fig 3-20c Three castings cleaned and ready for porcelain application (50 μm aluminum oxide and steam bath). The exercise will include one restoration on the maxillary right central incisor, two on the left lateral incisor, and two on the right canine using six different methods for duplicating CTC.

Table 3-1 Maverick over opaque technique

Hue-chroma	A3-3 (3 parts A3 + 1 part neutral)
Maverick	LB-4 (1 part light brown + 4 parts neutral)
Value	Enamel (high value)

	Firing order	Content	Remarks
1.	Opaque layer (thin wash)	A3 opaque	• Thin application covers approximately 50% of underlying metal color • Firing temperature — prescribed for opaque
2.	Porcelain margin (optional)		
3.	Transition layer (O-B-M)	Approximately ⅓ A3 opaque ⅓ A3 dentin ⅓ LB-4 (modifier)	• A mixture of opaque, dentin, and modifier is applied over the opaque wash • Surface is roughened while still in a semiwet state • Firing temperature — 10° lower than opaque wash • Underlying metal color should be eliminated upon completion of this firing
4.	First body porcelain layer	1 part light brown body modifier plus 4 parts neutral porcelain	• Uniformly cover entire transition layer with a thin layer of LB-4 (maverick dimension) • Completed firing should compare favorably with LB-4 customized shade tab
5.	Second body porcelain layer	3 parts A3 1 part neutral porcelain	• Build restoration to almost full contour, leaving enough room for enamel porcelain • Begin primary contour in semiwet porcelain
6.	Enamel layer	Enamel porcelain (high value)	• Cover entire restoration; build to full contour • Incorporate needed texture
7.	Glaze		• Fire to desired glaze or hand polish porcelain

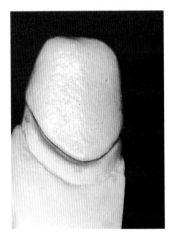 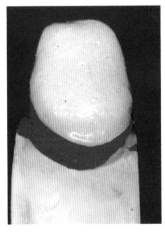 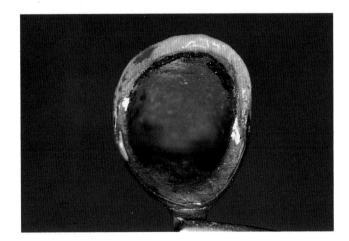

Fig 3-21a   **Fig 3-21b**   **Fig 3-21c**

Fig 3-21a Thin opaque wash (A3) fired to maxillary right central incisor using the maverick-over-opaque method for duplicating CTC. This layer should be almost too thin to measure, its main purpose being to mask approximately 50% of the underlying metal color. When a porcelain margin is included in the restoration, the opaque need not be extended onto the shoulder.

Fig 3-21b Porcelain margin fired to the shoulder of the die after the opaque wash. The slightly lower firing temperature of the porcelain margin material prevents any disturbance to the previously fired opaque. A second firing is usually required to compensate for shrinkage. The red indicator on the shoulder of the die highlights high spots on the margin that might prevent the casting from seating perfectly on the die.

Fig 3-21c Red indicator shows a high spot that prevents the casting from seating perfectly on the die. All high spots must be removed to obtain an acceptable marginal seal. To remove these high spots, a very fine diamond bur is used at slow speed to prevent possible chipping of the porcelain margin.

Maverick Over Opaque (Table 3-1)

Tooth enamel, with its fiberoptic-like characteristics, is able to transmit a small spot of maverick color, found in the dentin uniformly through the crown of the tooth. Enamel porcelain does not have this ability. Other means must be taken to duplicate the CTC that is evenly distributed over the entire tooth. One possible way to accomplish this with ceramics is to apply the color over the entire restoration. The duplicating method prescribed for this is "maverick over opaque." A thin layer of body modifier maverick dimension is applied over the the transition layer and fired. This will eventually influence the entire restoration uniformly, much like the tooth enamel is capable of doing with a spot of color directly beneath it (Figs 3-21a to l).

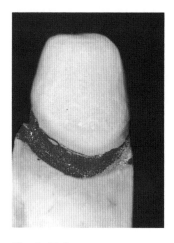

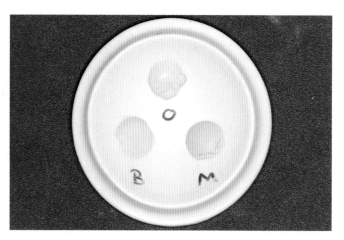

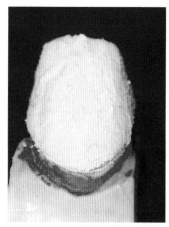

Fig 3-21d   **Fig 3-21e**   **Fig 3-21f**

Fig 3-21d   Porcelain margin seated on the die. The seal should pass a microscopic examination before the porcelain fabrication is begun. If the examination shows an incomplete seal, another application of margin material must be fired to fill the voids. The firing temperature for each subsequent firing should be lowered 5°. Once a perfect seal has been obtained, the labial surface of the margin material is chamfered to create space for the transition layer.

Fig 3-21e   Measured portions of material that make up the transition layer: equal portions of opaque, body (dentin), and body modifier (maverick dimension). In this exercise, the body (hue-chroma) will be A3-3; maverick dimension, LB-4. The transition layer will therefore consist of one third opaque A3, one third dentin A3-3, and one third body modifier LB-4. This is mixed with distilled water to a pasty consistency and made ready for the next application. Portions of each component can be varied to meet the needs of the restoration.

Fig 3-21f   A transition layer is applied over the previously fired opaque wash and porcelain margin material. The pasty consistency of the mixture promotes a textured surface, which is necessary to diffuse color and light. The chamfered porcelain margin permits complete coverage of the transition layer. Before the transition layer is fired, any porcelain that might have seeped onto the inner surface of the porcelain margin must be removed.

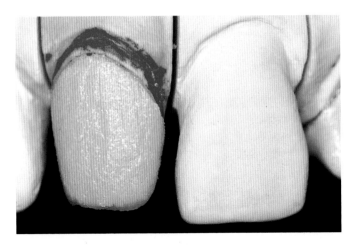

Fig 3-21g The fired transition layer displays a textured surface that will help create a more lifelike restoration. The transition layer is probably the most important ingredient of the entire restoration in that the hue-chroma and maverick color dimensions have been placed deep into the restoration, with the thickness of metal, opaque, and transition layer measuring only approximately 0.25 mm. The firing temperature of the transition layer is 10° below that of the porcelain margin material. At this point, there should be no color influence from the metal substructure.

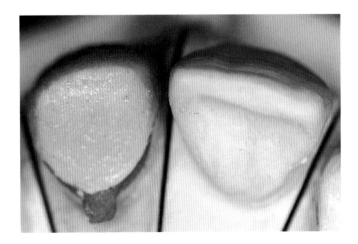

Fig 3-21h At this stage of porcelain fabrication, even though the labial aspect of the restoration is almost in line with the left central incisor, the CTC has already been established and the remaining 0.75-mm available space is sufficient room for dentin and enamel. The firing temperature of the transition layer is 10° higher than that of dentin and enamel because of the small amount of opaque in the mixture. The textured surface will thus not melt into the dentin but will remain during the dentin and enamel firing.

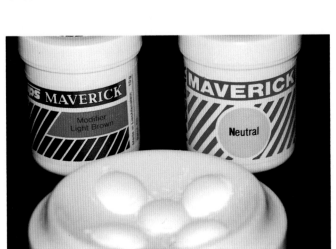

Fig 3-21i Porcelain mixing palette with measured portions of maverick dimension LB-4 (one part light brown body modifier and four parts neutral porcelain). The Maverick Porcelain System kit supplies premixed shades, which eliminates the need to measure. Either buildup liquid or distilled water is used in the mixture, which is spatulated to a creamy consistency, not the paste used in the transition layer.

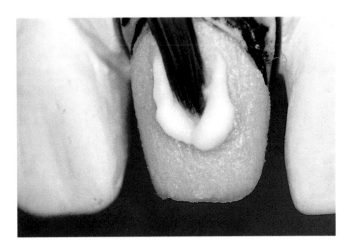

Fig 3-21j In the maverick-over-opaque duplicating method, a thin application of the maverick dimension (LB-4) is brushed over the transition layer, taking care to fill in its rough surface. If not properly applied, air could become trapped, resulting in porosity and/or expanded air pockets during firing. This could eventually cause a fracture. This application must be slightly condensed.

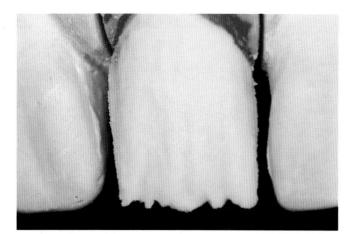

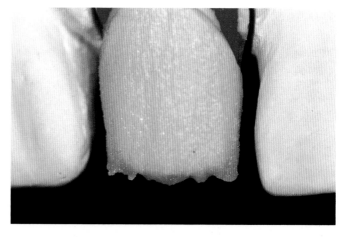

Fig 3-21k The creamy mixture of LB-4 is distributed evenly over the entire transition layer, keeping the thickness to a minimum (0.05 mm). At this stage, the incisal edge is contoured to mask the underlying crescent shape of the casting. An incisal matrix can be used to show the remaining available room for dentin and enamel porcelain. The firing temperature is 10° lower than that of the transition layer, thus preventing the rough texture from melting away.

Fig 3-21l Fired maverick dimension (LB-4) displays a color influence evenly distributed over the entire restoration. The rough surface of the transition layer has survived the firing and will remain throughout the entire fabrication of the restoration. This firing typifies the maverick-over-opaque method in that this layer will influence the restoration uniformly. At this stage, the thickness of metal, opaque wash, transition layer, and maverick dimension should measure approximately 0.3 mm.

The next porcelain layer is the hue-chroma dimension, which is made up of either the hue selection (fully concentrated) or chroma, a diluted version of the hue. At this point, three of the four tooth color dimensions have been incorporated into the restoration (Figs 3-22a to d). It is now covered with enamel porcelain, which regulates the brightness (value) of the colors as they project through it. Normally it is thicker in the incisal/buccal third and becomes progressively thinner toward the gingival third, permitting more color to show through. The light passes through the enamel and dentin and strikes the roughened layer, where it picks up color in the transition layer. The rough surface helps diffuse the light, carrying with it these deeply embedded colors. These colors join with the maverick color covering the transition layer, along with the colors incorporated in the dentin, and project through the enamel porcelain (Figs 3-23a and b).

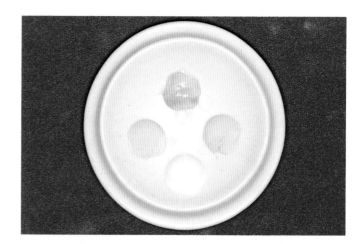

Fig 3-22a Dentin (hue-chroma dimension A3-3) is measured to proper proportions (three parts body porcelain A3 to one part neutral). The hue is desaturated by regulating parts of body porcelain to one part of neutral (the subnumber indicates the parts of body porcelain). Buildup liquid or distilled water is used in this mixture.

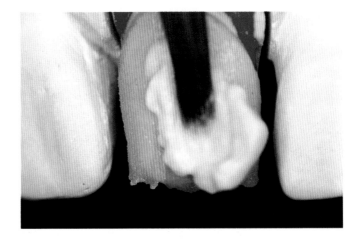

Fig 3-22b A creamy mixture of dentin (hue-chroma dimension) is applied over the maverick dimension. Slight condensation may be necessary to ensure an even, dense, porous-free layer of color. Adequate condensing in each stage is important because of the ultrathin applications. The closer the color particles are vibrated together, the more effect they will have in reproducing true CTC.

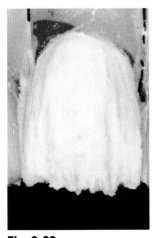

Fig 3-22c

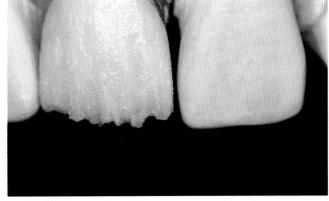

Fig 3-22d

Fig 3-22c Completed dentin layer buildup with slightly overbuilt interproximal and incisal areas to compensate for shrinkage. Some shrinkage is desirable to allow room for enamel porcelain. During this stage, the incisal edge should be contoured much like that established during the maverick application. Provisions should be made during this stage to create a transparent incisal edge, if indicated.

Fig 3-22d Fired dentin. At this point, three of the four tooth color dimensions have been layered into the restoration; hue-chroma and maverick. Note the shrinkage, which creates room for enamel porcelain and obviates the need to grind. With any grinding in delicate layering techniques such as this, there is the danger of removing needed color. Each layer should therefore be applied accurately. The total thickness at this stage is approximately 0.6 mm.

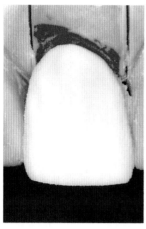

Fig 3-23a

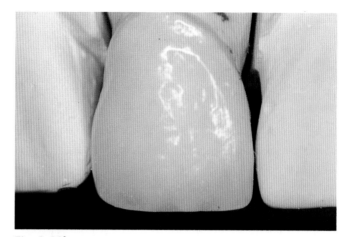

Fig 3-23b

Fig 3-23a Enamel application. Dentin is covered completely with enamel porcelain. The value dimension is assigned to the enamel of the natural tooth; the same assignment is made to the enamel porcelain of the restoration, even though they differ greatly in their physical and chemical makeup. The average thickness of natural enamel is 1 mm; the enamel porcelain of a ceramic restoration is 0.3 mm. It is slightly overbuilt to compensate for shrinkage.

Fig 3-23b The contoured and glazed maxillary right central incisor measures 0.9 mm, including metal, opaque, transition, maverick, dentin, and enamel layers. In the maverick-over-opaque method for duplicating CTC, the maverick dimension influences the restoration uniformly. Note the absence of areas of saturated color such as are found in the embedded maverick method.

The maverick over opaque method for duplicating CTC is recommended for restorations needing a subtle, even distribution of the maverick dimension with no visible areas of color concentration. The thin maverick covering also helps to diminish the opaque effect by lowering its value.

Embedded Maverick (Table 3-2)

Unlike the maverick over opaque duplicating method, which is used where uniform color is needed in a restoration, the embedded maverick method is used when color accents are required in certain areas, such as when teeth have spots of maverick color that are concentrated enough to show through the enamel layer quite noticeably. Even though the entire tooth is somewhat influenced by this spot of maverick color, its location is obvious and can be seen projecting through the enamel. These accent areas can be located in any section of the tooth, for no apparent reason, thus the term maverick color.

In natural teeth, even though there is no set rule or pattern as to where the maverick colors are located, color family is usually uniform (that is, seldom, if ever, will you find the yellow maverick family in the same arch as orange or light brown).

Table 3-2   Embedded maverick technique

Firing order	Content	Remarks
1. Opaque layer (thin wash)	A3 opaque	• Thin application covers approximately 50% of underlying metal color • Firing temperature — prescribed for opaque
2. Transition layer (O-B-M)	Approximately 1/3 A3 opaque 1/3 A3 dentin 1/3 LB-4 (modifier)	• A mixture of opaque, dentin, and modifier is applied over the opaque wash • Surface is roughened while still in a semiwet state • Firing temperature — 10° lower than opaque wash • Underlying metal color should be eliminated upon completion of this firing
3. First body porcelain layer buildup with embedded maverick color	3 parts A3 1 part neutral plus 1 part light brown body modifier & 4 parts neutral	• Build up dentin (A3-3 + LB-4) to full contour allowing room for enamel porcelain • Scoop out areas of needed concentrated color and replace with maverick color (LB-4) and white modifier while still in semiwet state
4. Enamel layer	Enamel porcelain (high value)	• Cover entire restoration; build to full contour • Exact texturing in semiwet enamel porcelain before firing • Optional — combine this step with first body porcelain layer
5. Glaze		• Natural glaze or hand polish

When a maverick color is detected, it is more important to determine the exact color family than its exact location or concentration. Color saturation varies from tooth to tooth; this makes it unnecessary to duplicate color concentration exactly.

The first step in duplicating CTC using the embedded maverick method is to build to full contour while leaving enough room for enamel porcelain. The body buildup consists of the hue-chroma dimension using the degree of saturation selected for the restoration. The areas in the restoration that need maverick deposits are scooped out and filled with the maverick color that was detected in the tooth (one portion of body modifier to the prescribed portions of neutral porcelain). These areas of maverick color should fill the scooped out area completely with no dentin cover while the body buildup is still in a semi-wet state (Figs 3-24a to i). The entire restoration is covered with enamel porcelain that has been mixed to the needed value (one large portion of enamel to small portions of gray modifier for low value and white modifier for high value). This places the embedded maverick color directly beneath the enamel porcelain layer, permitting it to project through the enamel unobstructed (Figs 3-25a and b).

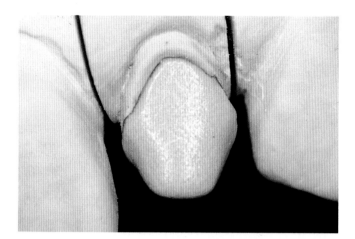

Fig 3-24a Thin opaque wash (A3) fired to the casting of the maxillary left lateral incisor, combining two methods for duplicating CTC: maverick plus hue-chroma and embedded maverick. This wash masks at least 50% of the underlying metal color and forms the beginning of CTC of the restoration. It also acts to degas the substructure by permitting gases to escape through its thin layer, which could otherwise cause porosity throughout the entire restoration.

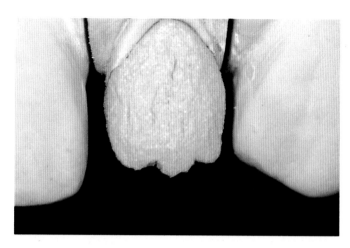

Fig 3-24b Transition layer combining opaque, body porcelain, and body modifier. Internal mamelons can be formed in the transition layer while the incisal edge is contoured. A porcelain margin will not be incorporated into this restoration, therefore the transition layer must be extended to cover the metal labial margin.

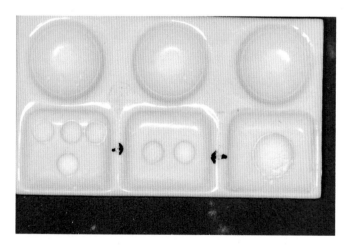

Fig 3-24c Measured portions of porcelain that will make up the body buildup (dentin) using the maverick plus hue-chroma method for duplicating CTC. One portion of body porcelain on the left (three parts A3 and one part neutral) and one portion of the body modifier on the right (premixed LB-4) are placed into the center well. The premixed body modifier found in the Maverick Porcelain System consists of one part light brown modifier and four parts neutral porcelain.

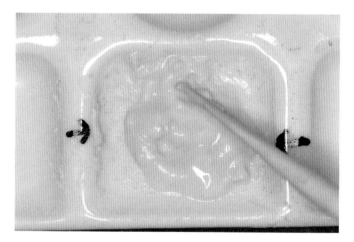

Fig 3-24d Buildup liquid or distilled water is added to the porcelain and spatulated thoroughly. The resultant mixture contains three parts A3 body porcelain, one part light brown modifier, and five parts neutral porcelain, thus combining the hue-chroma and maverick dimensions. This method for duplicating CTC works well on restorations that have insufficient space for layering these dimensions separately.

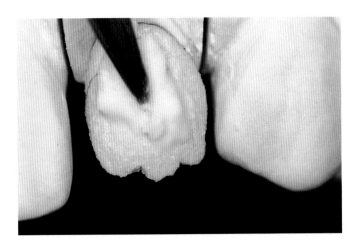

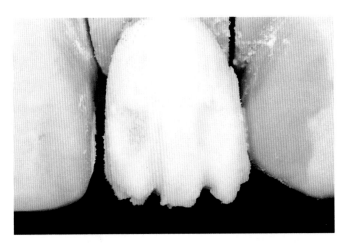

Fig 3-24e Body porcelain (dentin) is applied over the transition layer and condensed slightly to prevent trapping air onto the textured surface. This layer of porcelain should cover the transition layer completely, extending to the metal margin, keeping in mind that the embedded maverick method will be included in this restoration.

Fig 3-24f Body buildup completed with two scooped-out areas to accommodate embedded maverick colors. The embedded maverick method is used when CTC displays pronounced color deposits in certain areas of the tooth (ie, gingival third, interproximal area, incisal third). In this exercise, the maverick will be embedded labially in two areas.

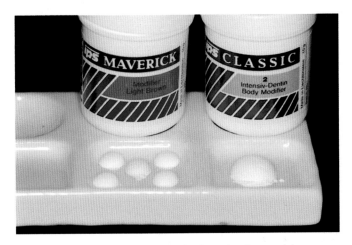

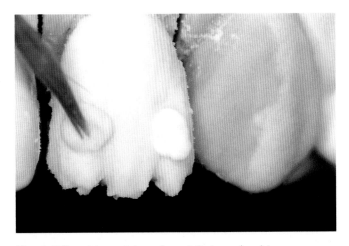

Fig 3-24g Light brown and white body modifiers are being prepared for embedding into the body buildup. One part light brown body modifier and four parts neutral porcelain will make up the embedded maverick for the scooped-out area mesially; white body modifier will be used distally. When selecting body modifiers for this method, only those that match the coefficient of expansion of the porcelain system should be considered.

Fig 3-24h Maverick colors LB-4 and white are embedded into the body buildup of the restoration. The body buildup must remain in a semiwet state while these modifiers are incorporated. Porcelain buildup done under dry conditions increases the likelihood that liquid will be pulled from the modifiers, resulting in porosity and/or a fracture. Gentle condensation will incorporate the modifiers into the body porcelain.

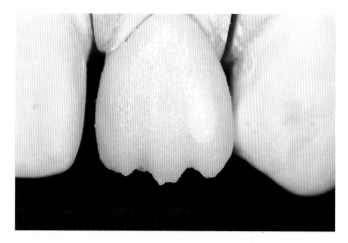

Fig 3-24i Fired dentin with visible embedded maverick colors. Note proper shrinkage to allow for the enamel layer with no excess porcelain to grind away. When areas of color are obvious in certain locations, the embedded maverick method should be considered. Location, color family, and concentration must be noted. Either a customized maverick shade guide or one supplied in the Maverick Porcelain System kit will meet these needs.

Maverick Buildup (Table 3-3)

The principle behind the maverick buildup method for duplicating CTC is the same as for embedded maverick except that in this method, the maverick colors are buried deeper into the restoration, thus projecting through the enamel in a more subtle fashion. This is accomplished by firing the spots of color directly over the transition layer. These spots of color are then covered with a layer of dentin and enamel porcelain. With this method, the maverick colors are almost undetectable, while still influencing CTC (Figs 3-26a to e).

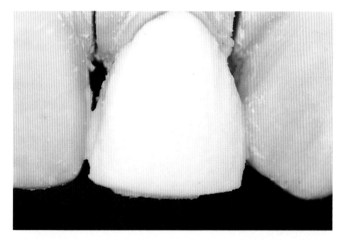

Fig 3-25a A high-value enamel porcelain is applied over the fired dentin. Even though the enamel layer is thin, it will regulate the brightness of the underlying colors as they are projected through it. The transition layer functions similarly to the enamel of the natural tooth. Light penetrates the thin enamel and dentin layers of the restoration, striking the rough surface of the transition layer, which reflects back to the eye (in a diffused fashion) all of the color dimensions contained in it.

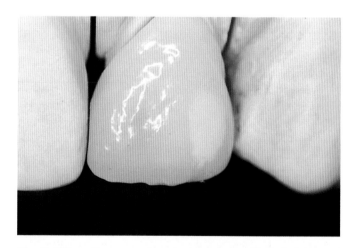

Fig 3-25b Contoured and glazed maxillary left lateral incisor restoration using a combination of two duplicating methods: maverick plus hue-chroma and embedded maverick. The embedded maverick method differs from the maverick-over-opaque (transition layer) method. The maverick dimension is concentrated in certain areas of the tooth in the former method whereas in the latter, it influences the tooth color uniformly. Duplicating methods can be used individually or in combination.

Table 3-3 Maverick buildup technique

Firing order	Content	Remarks
1. Opaque layer (thin wash)	A3 opaque	• Thin application covers approximately 50% of underlying metal color • Firing temperature — prescribed for opaque
2. Transition layer (O-B-M)	Approximately ¹/₃ A3 opaque ¹/₃ A3 dentin ¹/₃ LB-4 (modifier)	• A mixture of opaque, dentin, and modifier is applied over the opaque wash • Surface is roughened while still in a semiwet state • Firing temperature — 10° lower than opaque wash • Underlying metal color should be eliminated upon completion of this firing
3. Body modifier buildup over transition layer	1 part light brown body modifier plus 4 parts neutral porcelain	• Spots of color (LB-4 and white modifier) are fired directly over transition layer in just the designated areas
4. Dentin buildup	3 parts A3 1 part neutral porcelain 1 part LB 4 parts neutral	• Cover the entire restoration with dentin porcelain (including maverick color deposits)
5. Enamel layer	Enamel porcelain (high value)	• Cover entire restoration; build to full contour • Incorporate needed texture • Optional — combine this step with dentin buildup
6. Glaze		• Fire to desired glaze or hand polish porcelain

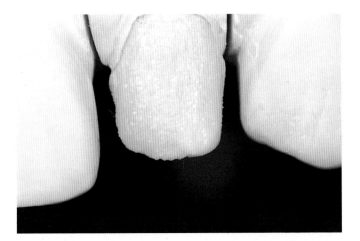

Fig 3-26a Two maverick colors (light brown [LB-4] and white) are fired directly over the transition layer in the maverick buildup method. This method is used when subtle maverick color concentrations are found in a tooth. The colors are placed deeper into the restoration as opposed to the embedded maverick method, where the colors are placed closer to the surface and are more pronounced.

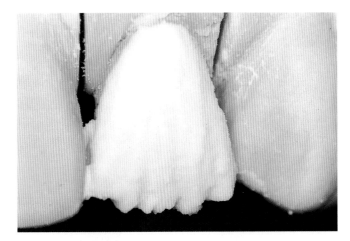

Fig 3-26b Dentin (hue-chroma A3-3) covers the transition layer and maverick deposits completely. The dentin layer helps obscure the effect of the maverick colors. Maverick buildup is usually the best method for duplicating this condition. Note the incisal scalloping to cover the underlying crescent shape of the casting.

111

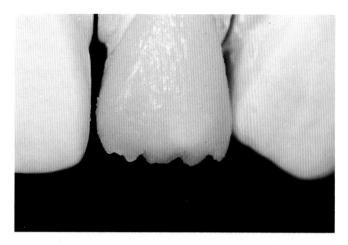

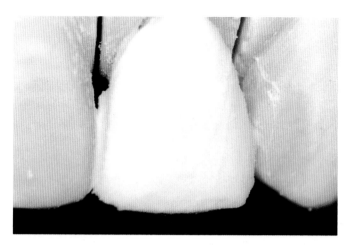

Fig 3-26c The fired dentin layer reveals subtle maverick deposits (LB-4 mesial; white distal). Although these deposits are almost unnoticeable in the mouth, the restoration will not harmonize with the surrounding natural teeth if they are not included. Attempting to apply these color deposits on the surface of the restoration with surface stains will often add to the problem and in most cases create an artificial appearance.

Fig 3-26d Dentin layer covered with enamel porcelain. At this stage, the maverick deposits have been covered by both the dentin and enamel, creating a subtle effect. In young patients who have tooth enamel with higher value than the porcelain system offers, a small portion of the white body modifier can be added to the enamel porcelain. When a lower-value enamel is required, small portions of gray body modifier can be added.

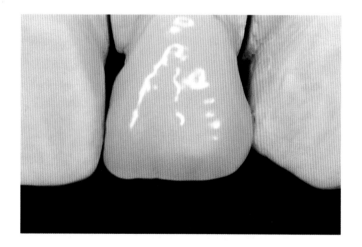

Fig 3-26e Contoured and glazed maxillary left lateral incisor using the maverick buildup method. The dentin and enamel covering layer makes it almost impossible to recognize this method, as compared to the embedded maverick method where the maverick deposits are placed closer to the surface and are covered only by enamel (see Fig 3-25b). The person determining the CTC should recognize the degree of subtlety and prescribe the most appropriate method.

Deep Stain Maverick (Table 3-4)

The deep stain maverick duplicating method is used for restoration with veneers that are so thin there is insufficient room for a body modifier. A stain is used in place of a modifier to supply the maverick dimension because it takes no thickness when applied directly onto the body buildup. This makes it possible to incorporate the four tooth color dimensions into a very thin veneer, like those often found in anterior restorations.

This method can be carried out in a single firing or several. The hue-chroma dimension is built over the transition layer to almost full contour, leaving room for enamel porcelain. Areas of needed maverick dimension, whether selective (as in embedded maverick) or uniformly over the entire dentin surface, are supplied by a stain that corresponds to the body modifier selected from the maverick shade guide.

Slight vibration is necessary to incorporate the stain liquid medium with the body buildup liquid. Also, care must be taken to keep internal staining at a minimum to prevent a change in the chemical makeup of the body porcelain. The slightest changes could interfere with the coefficient of expansion, resulting in porcelain fracture (Figs 3-27a and h).

Table 3-4 Deep stain maverick technique

	Firing order	Content	Remarks
1.	Opaque layer (thin wash)	A3 opaque	● Thin application covers approximately 50% of underlying metal color ● Firing temperature — prescribed for opaque
2.	Transition layer (O-B-M)	Approximately $\frac{1}{3}$ A3 opaque $\frac{1}{3}$ A3 dentin $\frac{1}{3}$ LB-4 (modifier)	● A mixture of opaque, dentin, and modifier is applied over the opaque wash ● Surface is roughened while still in a semiwet state ● Firing temperature — 10° lower than opaque wash ● Underlying metal color should be eliminated upon completion of this firing
3.	First body buildup	3 parts A3 1 part neutral porcelain thin layer light brown stain	● Build to full contour, leaving room for enamel coverage ● The stain is gently vibrated into the semiwet body porcelain; it corresponds to the body modifier selected for the maverick dimension
4.	Enamel layer	Enamel porcelain (high value)	● Cover entire restoration; build to full contour ● Incorporate needed texture ● Optional — combine this step with dentin buildup
5.	Glaze		● Fire to desired glaze or hand polish porcelain

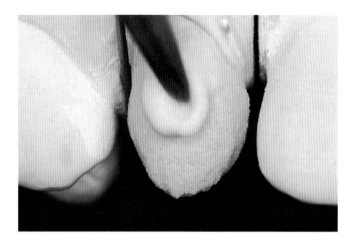

Fig 3-27a Dentin is applied over the fired transition layer of a maxillary right canine using the deep stain maverick method. This method, like the maverick plus hue-chroma method, is prescribed for restorations with a limited space for porcelain. The hue-chroma dimension is contained in the dentin. Distilled water is preferred over buildup liquid for the deep stain maverick method.

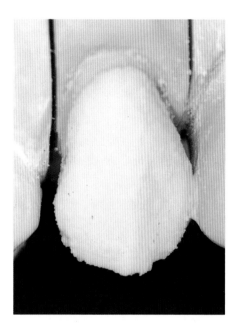

Fig 3-27b The body buildup has been completed. When porcelain layering is impractical because of lack of space, the dentin layer will be quite thin. However, at this stage, the presence of the hue-chroma dimension and the influence from the underlying transition layer make up for the minimal space. The added neutral porcelain to form the chroma dimension (A3-3) makes the transition layer even more effective.

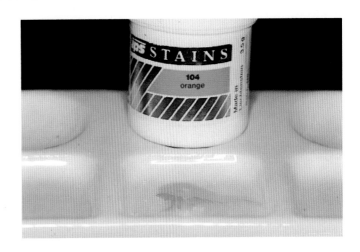

Fig 3-27c Stain selection to be used for deep stain maverick method. It must match the maverick dimension needed for CTC (LB-4). Stains are more potent than body modifiers, therefore care must be taken to dilute its strength to meet color requirements. Stain liquid medium is used rather than distilled water because of its ability to better suspend the color oxides. The amount of stain liquid medium determines the strength of the stain while maintaining the same color family.

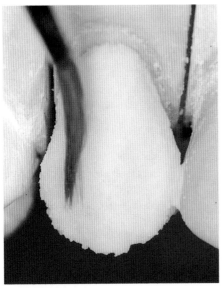

Fig 3-27d

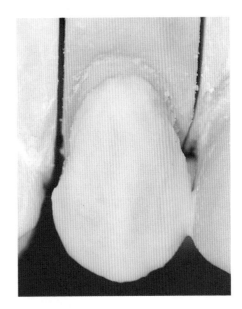

Fig 3-27e

Fig 3-27d Stain 104 is applied evenly over the body buildup (dentin). Stain can produce the same effect as body modifier but with no thickness. Internal staining requires certain precautions, the most important being the amount used. Excessive amounts could alter the coefficient of expansion of the dentin porcelain, which could cause fractures. Stain must be used sparingly.

Fig 3-27e The maverick dimension is incorporated into the prefired semiwet dentin (hue-chroma) with the use of stain rather than body modifier. The surface is covered uniformly with the stain, which must be gently condensed so that the stain liquid medium (a mixture of glycerin and water) can mix thoroughly with the distilled water in the body buildup. Otherwise, porosity could result.

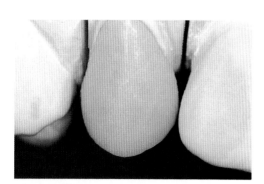

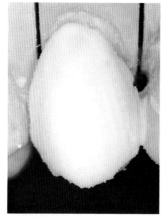

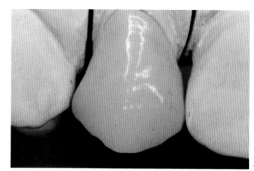

Fig 3-27f

Fig 3-27g

Fig 3-27h

Fig 3-27f Fired dentin that, even though rather thin, contains three color dimensions: hue, chroma, and maverick. It would have been difficult to accomplish this without the use of internal staining. Accurate buildup thickness is especially important in the deep stain maverick method because of the importance of firing shrinkage. Any needed reduction would remove the maverick dimension. Note sufficient shrinkage for the enamel layer.

Fig 3-27g Prefired enamel porcelain after full-contour buildup. Despite this thin layer, the enamel will regulate the brightness of the underlying color. The surface of the transition layer retains its rough surface during the entire fabrication and has much the same effect as natural enamel has with its fiberoptic capabilities.

Fig 3-27h Contoured and glazed maxillary canine using the deep stain maverick method. With this method, all four color dimensions can be included in restorations with limited space for porcelain. Internal staining plays a major role in dental ceramics, not only in restorations such as this, but also for reproducing irregularities found in natural dentition (see chapter 4).

Table 3-5 Maverick plus hue-chroma technique

Firing order	Content	Remarks
1. Opaque layer (thin wash)	A3 opaque	• Thin application covers approximately 50% of underlying metal color • Firing temperature — prescribed for opaque
2. Transition layer (O-B-M)	Approximately ⅓ A3 opaque ⅓ A3 dentin ⅓ LB-4 (modifier)	• A mixture of opaque, dentin, and modifier is applied over the opaque wash • Surface is roughened while still in a semiwet state • Firing temperature — 10° lower than opaque wash • Underlying metal color should be eliminated upon completion of this firing
3. Dentin buildup: mixture of maverick and hue-chroma	3 parts A3 5 parts neutral 1 part light brown body modifier	• Build to full contour, leaving room for enamel porcelain (cover completely)
4. Enamel porcelain application	Enamel porcelain (high value)	• Cover entire restoration with enamel porcelain • Incorporate needed anatomy, contour, and texture to minimize grinding • Enamel porcelain can be applied during body buildup
5. Glaze		• Natural glaze or hand polish

Maverick Plus Hue-Chroma (Table 3-5)

Another duplicating method that works well on restorations with thin veneers is maverick plus hue-chroma. In this method, the maverick and hue-chroma dimensions are mixed together and used as the dentin buildup material. The mixture is determined by the proportions of dentin, body modifier, and neutral porcelain found on customized color tabs that were used to measure the color dimensions in the prepared tooth. For example, if the hue-chroma dimension is A3-3 and the maverick dimension is LB-4, the body (dentin) buildup porcelain (hue-chroma) would be: three parts A3, one part neutral porcelain; maverick would be one part light brown body modifier, four parts neutral porcelain. The mixture would be three parts A3, one part light brown body modifier, and five parts neutral porcelain (the buildup material for the restoration). This is then covered completely with enamel porcelain (see Figs 3-24c to e).

Surface Maverick (Table 3-6)

Surface maverick is usually associated with worn incisal edges of anterior teeth. As the enamel wears away in this area, the dentin becomes exposed and vulnerable to discoloration. Discoloration begins incisally and will eventually engulf the entire dentin. While the dentin retains its hue-chroma dimension, giving way to discoloration only at the incisal edge, the best method for duplication is surface maverick.

The restoration is built to full contour with dentin and enamel. The incisal edge is scooped out and replaced with prescribed body modifier (maverick dimension). When more color is needed, stain is added to intensify to modifier (before firing) (Figs 3-28a and b).

A single unit should be duplicated exactly to blend with surrounding teeth. When restoring the entire six maxillary or mandibular anterior teeth, this method should be considered, the color intensity being determined by the patient's age and the

Table 3-6 Surface maverick technique

Firing order	Content	Remarks
1. Opaque layer (thin wash)	A3 opaque	• Thin application covers approximately 50% of underlying metal color • Firing temperature — prescribed for opaque
2. Transition layer (O-B-M)	Approximately ⅓ A3 opaque ⅓ A3 dentin ⅓ LB-4 (modifier)	• A mixture of opaque, dentin, and modifier is applied over the opaque wash • Surface is roughened while still in a semiwet state • Firing temperature — 10° lower than opaque wash • Underlying metal color should be eliminated upon completion of this firing
3. Dentin buildup: hue-chroma dimension	3 parts A3 1 part neutral	• Build dentin to almost full contour, leaving room for enamel porcelain
4. Enamel built to full contour	Enamel porcelain (high value)	• After building to full contour with enamel, scoop out incisal edge approximately 1 mm and fill with body modifier
Incisal edge: modified with maverick color	LB-4	• This step can be combined with step 3
5. Glaze		• Natural glaze or hand polish

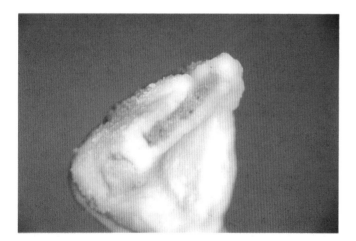

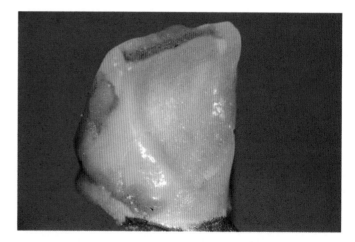

Fig 3-28a Surface maverick. The incisal edge of a prefired maxillary central incisor restoration is scooped out and filled with selected maverick color. Body modifier can usually fulfill this purpose, however when stronger colors are needed, stain can be added to body modifier to increase the intensity. Just as in porcelain layering, the porcelain buildup must be done in a semiwet state. Although gentle condensation is required to disperse color particles and liquid, care must be taken to maintain contour and not interfere with previously layered colors.

Fig 3-28b Restoration as it appeared after firing with no needed shaping. In this method, the dentin retains the hue-chroma dimension; only the exposed discolored dentin is altered. Dentin discoloration usually begins when enamel is worn away. The exposed porous dentin immediately begins to discolor, locally at first and eventually throughout. The two most common areas for enamel wear are the incisal edge and gingival third (gingival erosion). The surface maverick method is usually used in combination with one or several other of the seven methods.

Table 3-7 Maverick and enamel technique

	Firing order	Content	Remarks
1.	Thin opaque wash	Light brown opaque	• Thin opaque layer should cover approximately 50% of metal substructure color • Should be fired to maximum opaque maturing temperature
2.	Transition layer	Transition LB-4 Mixture of ¹/₂ opaque and ¹/₂ body modifier	• Surface should be roughened while porcelain is in a semiwet state • Firing temperature must be lowered approximately 15°
3.	Body buildup	(LB-4) 1 part light brown modifier 4 parts neutral porcelain	• Build restoration to full contour, leaving room for enamel porcelain
4.	Enamel application	Enamel LB	• Cover entire restoration with enamel porcelain • Incorporate needed contour and texture before firing • Enamel can be applied with body buildup (step 3)
5.	Glaze		• Natural furnace glaze or hand polish

condition of the remaining natural dentition. This gives the ceramist an opportunity to incorporate natural color and contour typical for the patient's oral health.

Maverick and Enamel (Table 3-7)

Incisal wear and/or age could eventually cause the entire dentin to discolor completely. Discoloration can progress until the dentin color is out of range of normal tooth color (hue-chroma dimension) and into the maverick color range. The maverick color guide is then needed for detecting and measuring the maverick dimension and is the only possible method for duplicating would-be maverick and enamel. In this method, we are concerned with just two dimensions: maverick and value. The entire body buildup is made with the prescribed body modifier (maverick dimension) and covered completely with the prescribed enamel porcelain (value dimension).

Being out of the color range of the common commercial shade guide, alterations must be made in the opaque layer. It must correspond to the basic color family of the body modifier (yellow, orange, light brown, and dark brown).

The opaque layer consists of opaque from the basic color family. The transition layer is made up of 50% of the same opaque and 50% body modifier selected for the restoration.

The body buildup is made with modifiers, satisfying the maverick dimension, then is covered completely with enamel porcelain. (Figs 3-29a to l).

A porcelain system designed especially to comply with the needs of the maverick and enamel duplicating method is available in the United

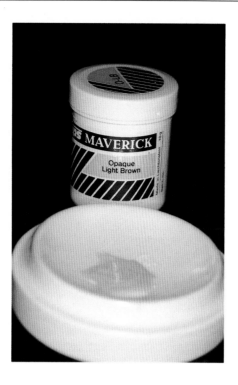

Fig 3-29a Premixed opaque contained in the Maverick Porcelain System used specifically in the maverick-and-enamel method. The system contains four color families: yellow, honey yellow, light brown, and dark brown. Every maverick color found in the natural dentition can be duplicated with this porcelain system. The opaques are formulated to enhance the CTC by complementing the transition layer, dentin, and enamel.

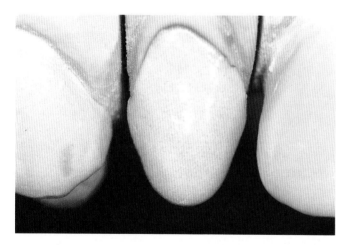

Fig 3-29b Light brown maverick opaque wash applied over metal casting. The opaque should mask at least 50% of the underlying metal color. Several applications may be needed to accomplish this with alloys that tend to darken greatly (ie, semiprecious and nonprecious). CTC of a restoration begins in the opaque layer. To obtain optimum results, the opaque must comply with the needs of the other porcelain layers.

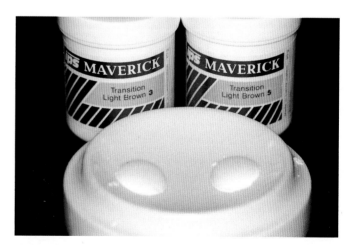

Fig 3-29c Premixed transition porcelain used for the maverick and enamel duplicating method. The maverick dimension in this exercise is LB-4. Equal parts of T-LB-3 and T-LB-5 make up T-LB-4. This is mixed with distilled water to a thick consistency, keeping in mind that it must form a textured surface over the opaque wash.

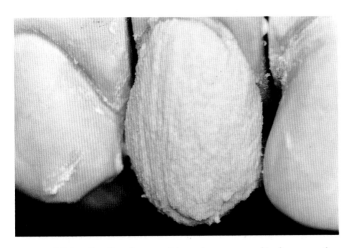

Fig 3-29d Prefired transition layer applied over the opaque wash, leaving a textured surface. In restorations that require concentrated color in certain areas (eg, gingival erosion, interproximal areas), these colors can be incorporated into the transition layer at this stage. Body modifiers must be used for this purpose; the color oxides in stain do not survive the maturing temperature of the transition porcelain.

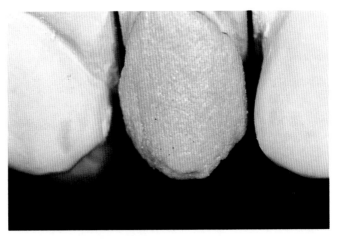

Fig 3-29e Fired transition layer, which has retained a textured surface. The degree of texture will vary with the thickness of the restoration. With restorations less than 3/4 mm, the surface must be textured less, to prevent areas of transition porcelain from protruding through the fired dentin layer. Even a finely textured transition layer can diffuse color and light in much the same way as natural enamel. Note that the canine contour has been established at this stage.

Fig 3-29f Premixed body porcelain (dentin). LB-4 can be created in two ways: (1) by combining equal portions of B-LB-3 and B-LB-5, and (2) by adding four parts of neutral porcelain to one part of M-LB (fully saturated light brown body modifier). Either mixture will produce the same result. Buildup liquid or distilled water can be used with both.

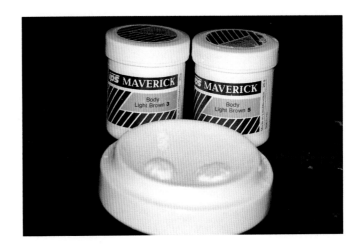

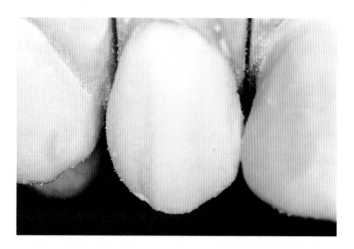

Fig 3-29g Prefired body buildup (LB-4) following the basic contour established during the transition stage. Dentin is built to almost full contour, allowing for shrinkage and space for enamel. In ultrathin restorations, much of the CTC is derived from the transition layer.

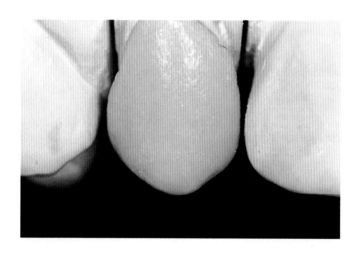

Fig 3-29h The fired dentin layer displays the selected color (LB-4). The resultant color to this point is created by the combined effects of opaque, transition layer, and body porcelain. At this stage, the color should match perfectly with the dentin of the prepared tooth. It is obvious that the dentin has discolored to the degree that it is out of the range of the hue-chroma customized shade guide. Either a maverick customized shade guide or one supplied with the Maverick Porcelain System must be used.

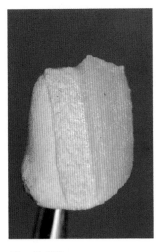

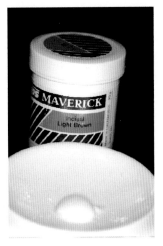

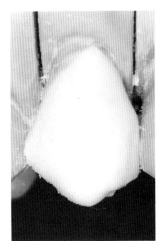

Fig 3-29i

Fig 3-29j

Fig 3-29k

Fig 3-29i Fired layers of porcelain supplied in the Maverick Porcelain System show the effect each has on CTC before application of the enamel porcelain. Each layer is fired with subsequently lower temperatures so that each previous layer is unaltered. This is particularly important for the transition layer. Note that even after the dentin has been fired, the surface of the transition layer has maintained its textured surface, which is necessary to diffuse and reflect color with the light that has penetrated the enamel and dentin layers.

Fig 3-29j Enamel porcelain that has been formulated to complement the maverick dimension LB (light brown). The Maverick Porcelain System has premixed enamels (incisals) for each color family: yellow, honey yellow, light brown, and dark brown. Each is designed to supply the proper value to regulate brightness as the color dimensions pass through it. Buildup liquid or distilled water is used for mixing.

Fig 3-29k The restoration is slightly overbuilt with enamel LB to cover the entire dentin, just as is found in natural dentition. When duplicating dentition, it is important to recognize not only the chemical makeup, such as color and organic and inorganic substances, but also physical properties such as component location. Enamel is often overlooked. It covers the entire crown of the tooth, therefore it should cover the entire restoration, not just the incisal one third, as is commonly found.

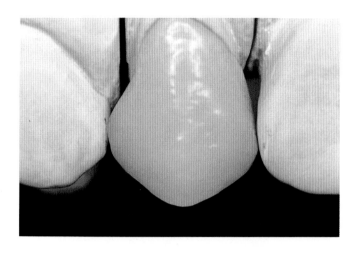

Fig 3-29l Contoured and glazed maxillary right canine restoration using the maverick and enamel method. This method differs from the surface maverick method in that the entire dentin of the tooth has darkened, while in the surface maverick the dentin still falls within the hue-chroma dimension with the maverick dimension visible only in areas where the dentin is unprotected by enamel. Surface maverick will eventually develop into the maverick and enamel category.

Table 3-8 "No maverick" technique

	Firing order	Content	Remarks
1.	Thin opaque wash	A3 opaque	• Covers 50% of underlying metal color
2.	Transition layer	1 part A3 opaque 1 part (A3-3) body porcelain	• A mixture of approximately ½ each of opaque and body porcelain • Roughen surface before firing, while still in semiwet state • Firing temperature: 15° below opaque wash
3.	Body buildup	3 parts A3 body porcelain 1 part neutral porcelain	• Build restoration to almost full contour, leaving room for enamel
4.	Enamel layer	Enamel porcelain (high value)	• Cover entire restoration; build to full contour • Incorporate needed contour and texture before firing • Enamel can be applied with body buildup (step 3)
5.	Glaze		• Fire to desired glaze or hand polish

States and Europe. The Maverick Porcelain System includes premixed opaques, transition powders, dentin, and enamel porcelains.

No Maverick (Table 3-8)

In some teeth, we find no maverick dimension, especially in young patients. In cases such as this, the concern is only with the hue-chroma and value dimensions. The basic color (hue) is determined from the dentin and further refined with the chroma dimension. In the no maverick method, the body buildup (dentin) is made with either the hue or chroma selection. The opaque layer is a thin wash. The transition layer is composed of 25% opaque and 75% body porcelain. The body is built to full contour, leaving room for enamel por-

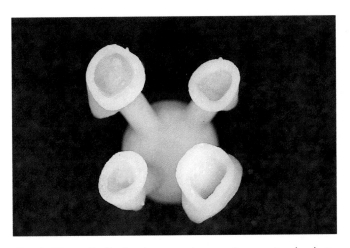

Fig 3-30a Deflasked ceramic castings attached to sprues. Casting is achieved with the combined efforts of vacuum and pressure. The castings are sprayed with glass beads (100 μm) at low pressure. They must be perfectly free of investment particles to prevent problems during porcelain fabrication. Note the ideal shoulder preparations over the entire circumference of the castings. This is necessary for sufficient strength and support for the restoration. The castings are now ready to be separated from the sprues and prepared for fabrication.

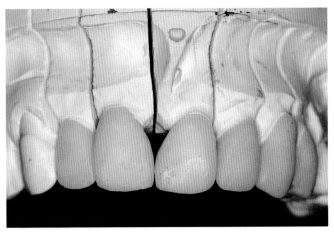

Fig 3-30b The casting is placed onto the master working model after being detached from the sprues. It is an exact duplicate of the original waxup. The case is waxed to either full or partial contour (depending on which fabricating technique will be used), invested, and cast. Here, the porcelain layering technique will be used, therefore a partial waxup was required to supply basic contour with no refinement. The castings will eventually be cut back to make room for porcelain. (The dentin color [hue dimension] has already been obtained in the casting.)

celain. This can be accomplished in two separate firings or in a single firing with both body and enamel.

Enamel Porcelain Application

Enamel porcelain can be applied with the dentin buildup or separately, after the dentin has been fired. Firing separately gives the ceramist an opportunity to make refinements in the fired dentin before enamel application. The incisal matrix will determine the exact amount of space available for enamel. If some areas are too bulky to allow for enamel, dentin reduction will be required.

Enamel porcelain covers the dentin while completely filling the incisal matrix. (It might be necessary to slightly overbuild incisally to compensate for shrinkage.)

If properly built up, only a minimal amount of contouring should be required. This is important because too much grinding can remove needed color.

The finished restoration should comply with both the incisal matrix and study model for acceptable function and esthetics.

Duplicating CTC in an All-Ceramic Restoration (Figs 3-30a to r)

For a color system to be successful, it must have the facilities to satisfy all mediums. In this exercise, the IPS Empress (Ivoclar, Liechtenstein; Williams Dental, Buffalo, NY) all-ceramic system will be used to show how the Four-Dimensional Tooth Color System can be used to duplicate CTC. The

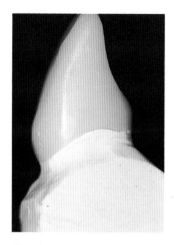 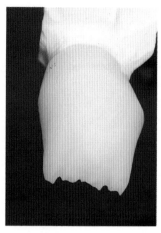 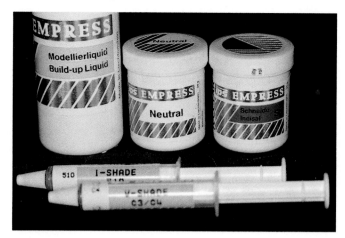

Fig 3-30c   **Fig 3-30d**   **Fig 3-30e**

Fig 3-30c   A leucite-reinforced ceramic casting before cutback displays a typical marginal seal. The IPS Empress ceramic system, with its unique casting system, produces excellent marginal seals. As with any other restoration, a well-constructed wax pattern, with emphasis on a perfect margin, is of prime importance. The chances of routinely obtaining these results using the Empress system are good.

Fig 3-30d   The ceramic casting is cut back to allow for porcelain. In the layering technique where the prescribed dentin color is present and no maverick dimension is involved, fabrication is uncomplicated. Enamel porcelain is applied over the cutback and fired, contoured, and glazed. Hue and value (not maverick) are the only color dimensions duplicated. If a chroma dimension is needed, a layer of neutral porcelain is fired between the enamel and dentin to dilute the strength of the hue.

Fig 3-30e   The IPS Empress System is simple and uncomplicated and supplies all the needed material to duplicate CTC. The absence of a metal substructure and the opaque layer needed to block out its color influence, leaves more space for porcelain and colorants. The basic porcelains for layering are neutral and enamel. Also included are stains and modifiers that are mixed with each to obtain optimum results.

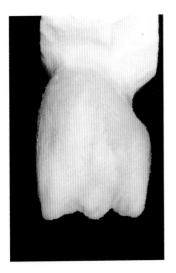
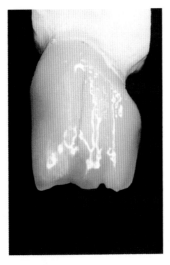
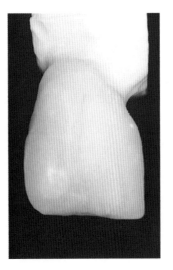
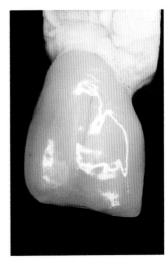

Fig 3-30f   **Fig 3-30g**   **Fig 3-30h**   **Fig 3-30i**

Fig 3-30f The first layer of porcelain is applied over the casting cutback. The cutback (see Fig 3-30d) should be designed to make room for embedded colors (embedded maverick and maverick buildup methods). These color modifiers are incorporated into the restoration during vertical layering of neutral porcelain. As in the case of metal ceramic restorations, the buildup must be semiwet while the modifiers and stains are placed. The hue dimension is present in the original casting, and the transition layer is unnecessary.

Fig 3-30g Fired porcelain buildup comprising hue-chroma and maverick dimensions. Also included are several subtle and bold irregularities: craze and check lines, interproximal and incisal discoloration, and hypocalcification (see chapter 4). Note the incisal edge contour, developed from the porcelain buildup (see Fig 3-30f) that covered the original incisal contour (see Fig 3-30d). The overlapping, contrasting incisal contours create a sense of depth.

Fig 3-30h The body buildup is covered completely with enamel porcelain, fired, and contoured for glaze. The enamel regulates the brightness of the underlying color dimensions. It also adds subtlety to the irregularities built into the sublayer of porcelain.

Fig 3-30i Glazed IPS Empress ceramic restoration using the porcelain layering technique. The four tooth color dimensions that make up the CTC along with several irregularities are quite obvious. The well-glazed full-circumference porcelain margin with its optimum seal presents a superb environment for gingival tissue management. When a restoration requires irregularities such as this, the layering technique is a better choice than the staining technique where the colors are painted on the surface of the ceramic casting.

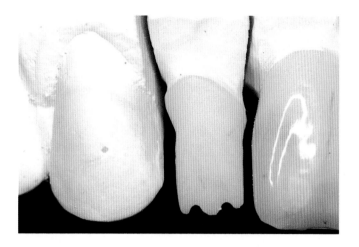

Fig 3-30j Contoured ceramic casting for a maxillary right lateral incisor. Note the eroded gingival area of the canine. The gingival area of the casting has been chamfered to harmonize with it. Also, mamelons have been contoured into the incisal third, leaving space for a more translucent incisal edge. In this exercise, the no-maverick method for duplicating CTC will be used for the middle third of the restoration; surface maverick will be used at the gingival third.

IPS Empress System is one of several available that is classified as being metal free. It employs the "lost-wax principle" to fabricate a leucite-reinforced ceramic that is said to have many qualities found in natural dentition. The system is capable of producing anterior and posterior restorations as well as inlays and onlays. Two techniques can be used: (1) layering and (2) staining.

Layering Technique

In the layering technique, dentin-colored ingots (in both Ivoclar and Vita shades) are cast and used to comply with the dentin (hue) of the tooth. The fully contoured casting is cut back and prepared for porcelain application. If the first dimension (hue) that has been established in the casting appears to be too concentrated to satisfy CTC, a layer of neutral porcelain is fired over the casting to dilute the hue, developing the second color dimension, chroma. The third color dimension, maverick, is built into the restoration by means of the seven methods for duplicating CTC, which have been discussed previously. The enamel layer that covers the entire restoration becomes the fourth dimension, value.

Staining Technique

The staining technique is prescribed for posterior full-coverage inlays and onlays. Colorless ingots are available in two degrees of opacity. In this technique, the restoration must be waxed to full contour. The color is achieved through surface staining.

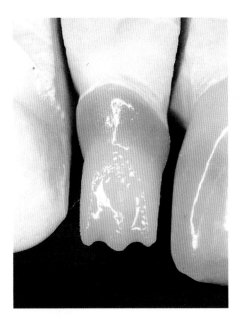 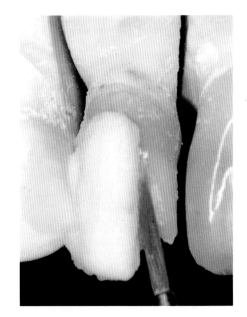

Fig 3-30k   **Fig 3-30l**

Fig 3-30k A mixture of neutral porcelain and stain is thoroughly mixed, applied to the gingival third of the casting, and fired. It is important to select the same color family found in the eroded area of the canine. A thin wash of neutral porcelain is fired over the remaining surface of the casting to ensure proper bonding of the body porcelain layer.

Fig 3-30l Vertical layering of neutral and enamel porcelain, incorporating several irregularities into the CTC. The gingival third surface maverick color was softened slightly to comply with a customized color tab that corresponded to the eroded canine. This can be done by thinning through grinding, as in this case, or by adding a layer of neutral porcelain. The eroded area is left exposed with no neutral covering (surface maverick method).

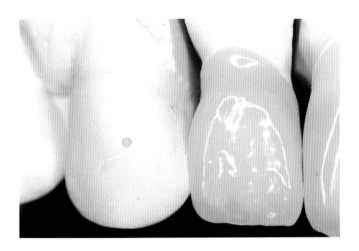

Fig 3-30m This contoured and glazed maxillary right lateral incisor emphasizes the importance of duplicating the contour and color of the eroded adjacent natural dentition. The all-ceramic restoration presents the technician with the opportunity to accomplish this even in a thin restoration. Also note the subtle craze lines, hypocalcification, mamelons, incisal translucency, and delicate incisal dentin frame (see chapter 4).

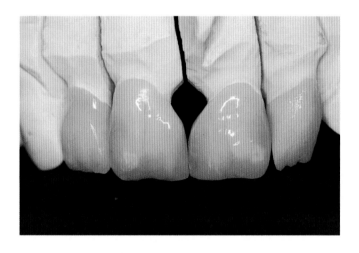

Fig 3-30n Three maxillary anterior incisors fabricated using the IPS Empress all-ceramic system (layering technique) compared to the ceramic casting of the left lateral incisor. Note how the basic family color of the casting prevails throughout the three completed restorations in spite of the color modifications necessary to include irregularities. This exercise illustrates how the Four Dimensional Tooth Color System is just as effective in duplicating CTC in an all-ceramic system as in a metal ceramic system.

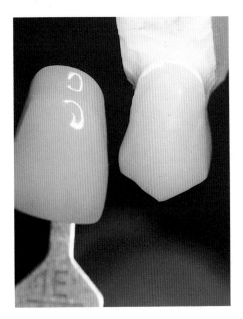

Fig 3-30o

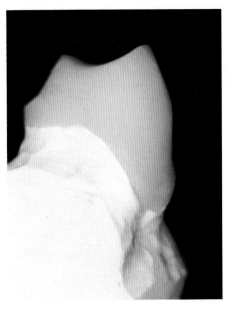

Fig 3-30p

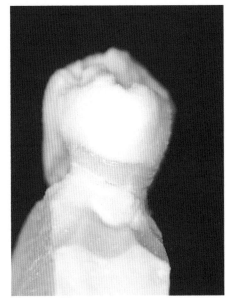

Fig 3-30q

Fig 3-30o   The family color of a premolar ceramic casting is compared with a color tab from the Chromascope, a tooth color guide included in the IPS Empress system. Even though the tab has an enamel layer, the family color is obvious enough to compare with that of the enamelless casting. Note the full contour of the casting, which gives the ceramist an opportunity to evaluate function and esthetics before fabrication with porcelain. If there is insufficient room occlusally for porcelain, centric stops should be included in the cast ceramic.

Fig 3-30p   Ceramic casting cut back to make room for neutral and enamel porcelains. The occlusal contour was added for support and strength. Although the cutback has reduced the thickness of the casting, the family color remains true (see Fig 3-30o). In fact, the material is so dense, it almost completely blocks out any color influence from cement or tooth structure. The advantage is that the family color of the finished restoration will be perceived the same in the mouth as on the master working cast.

Fig 3-30q   Prefired porcelain buildup over contoured premolar casting. Occlusal anatomy should be incorporated at this time to create a more natural-looking restoration. Right and left excursions will dictate the occlusal contour, while close attention is paid to premature contacts and lateral interferences. Note the 1-mm band of ceramic cast material throughout the entire circumference; this adds strength to the restoration and a foundation to build porcelain on.

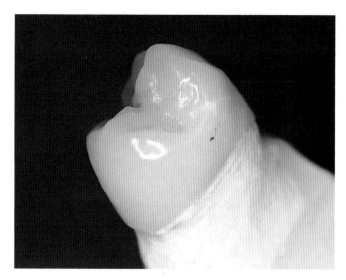

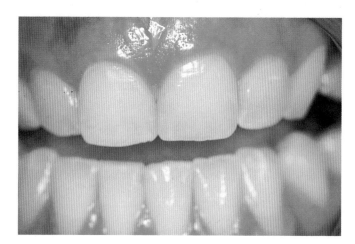

Fig 3-30r Glazed premolar restoration displaying many of the qualities found in natural dentition. The leucite-reinforced ceramic casting material is said to have the strength to withstand forces generated in the posterior region of the mouth. It combines its efforts with those of neutral and enamel porcelain that covers it, along with any needed color modifiers to project color and light in a very lifelike fashion. Note how well the porcelain combination blends with the cervical ceramic cast band.

Fig 3-31 Maxillary and mandibular arch, displaying information necessary to restore one or both maxillary central incisors. Family color and basic tooth form must be acknowledged while incorporating irregularities and modifications that harmonize with the remaining unrestored dentition. When restoring both incisors, some leeway is available. Restoration of just one incisor, however, requires more effort.

Maxillary Central Incisors (Figs 3-31 and 3-32a to k)

Of all the teeth in the mouth to be restored, the maxillary central incisors are probably of most concern, especially when only one incisor is involved. Most dentists and technicians will agree that the time and effort spent on a single central incisor often exceeds that spent on a full quadrant.

To help solve some of the problems involved with restoring one or both maxillary central incisors, you should be familiar with as many facts as possible surrounding their physical and chemical makeup. Only then can a more lifelike restoration be created.

When we discuss dental esthetics, our main concerns are color and contour, along with irregularities that harmonize with the surrounding unrestored dentition. Two basic rules are (1) adhere to family color, and (2) follow basic tooth form. This is especially true in the case of the maxillary central incisors. Without proper planning and evaluation, a restoration is recognized as such immediately.

Family Color

The same family color is usually found throughout the mouth. They can be classified into basic families, and every tooth has some degree of the same color except for color deformities or irregularities. Maxillary central incisors normally possess the same family color. This must be considered during restoration, especially when restoring only one incisor.

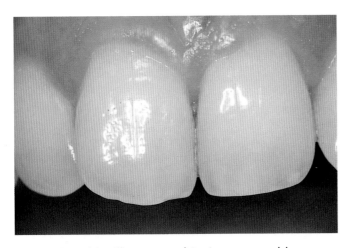

Fig 3-32a Maxillary central incisors are seldom symmetrical. Note the difference in overall shape. Also note the difference in the incisal contour, color concentration in the gingival and incisal thirds, and the very subtle interproximal color deposits.

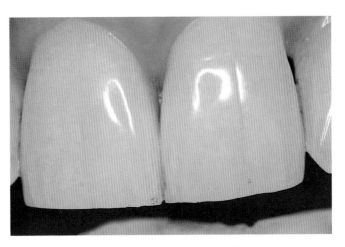

Fig 3-32b Slightly asymmetrical, maxillary central incisors, with interproximal color and differences in color concentration.

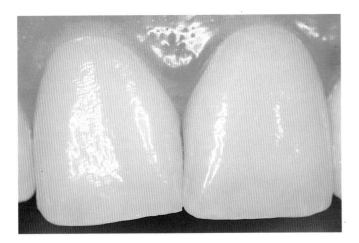

Fig 3-32c Differences in length of the maxillary central incisors are common. The difference can range from being slight to noticeable. Note the slightly longer left central incisor as compared to the right; both teeth, however, display the same degree of texture and glaze.

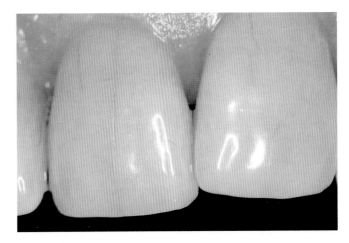

Fig 3-32d Malocclusion and lack of proper centric stops could cause noticeable length differences in the maxillary central incisors. If either is to be restored, function, not esthetics, should determine length. To change length during restoration without functional consideration could lead to failure. Also, note the higher concentration of color in the right central incisor and the subtle interproximal color.

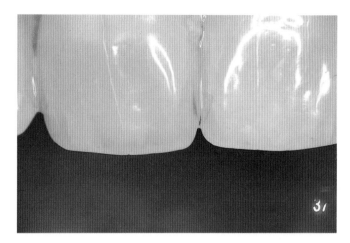

Fig 3-32e Note the difference in color concentration and location in the incisal third of the maxillary central incisors. In the restoration of a central incisor it is not necessary to copy the unrestored tooth exactly. Once the family color has been selected, concentration and location are not important.

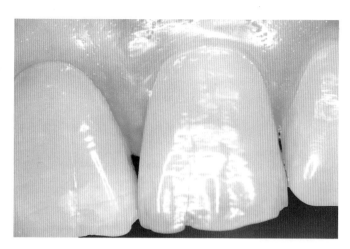

Fig 3-32f Left central incisor with deformed incisal edge. Irregularities are not always common to both maxillary central incisors. This holds especially true where color is concerned; craze and check lines, hypocalcification, color deposits, etc, are often found in one tooth and not the other. When restoring one or both teeth, therefore, subtle irregularities can be placed in either, with little regard to location or symmetry.

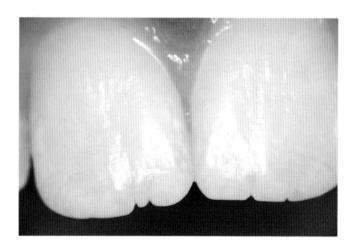

Fig 3-32g Maxillary central incisors displaying differences in incisal edge contour. This is common in natural dentitions. The incisal edge of the maxillary central incisors are usually the most visible portion of these teeth and much can be done to make the restoration more natural looking by purposely miscontouring it. Also, note the same degree of texture and glaze and subtle interproximal color.

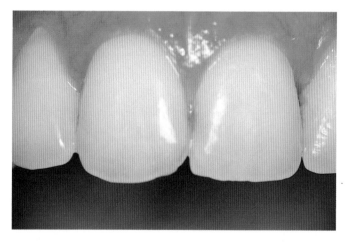

Fig 3-32h A pronounced difference in incisal edge position and contour between the maxillary central incisors is quite evident, while maintaining basic tooth form. Texture and glaze are conspicuously lacking on both teeth.

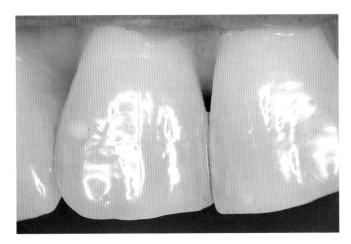

Fig 3-32i Age can contribute to length differences brought about by wear and supraeruption. Note hypocalcification spot on distal lobe of right central incisor and interproximal color.

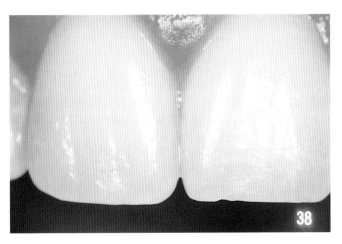

Fig 3-32j A textured labial surface can usually be associated with young teeth. When present, both maxillary central incisors exhibit the same degree; seldom is there a noticeable difference when comparing them. Note differences in incisal edge position and contour and very subtle interproximal color.

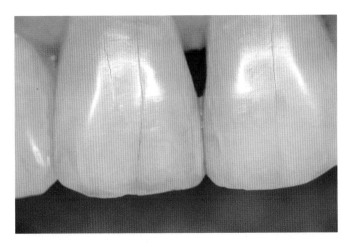

Fig 3-32k Surface texture lessens and sometimes disappears with age. Wear and eating habits help bring this about and do not necessarily affect the health of the tooth. Note interproximal color and incisal edge position and contour.

Basic Tooth Form

Tooth shape can be classified into three basic forms: square, ovoid, and tapering. The general shape of the maxillary central incisors can vary somewhat, but overall, the forms should coincide.

Along with fulfilling these fundamental requirements in color and contour, other characteristics must be pointed out.

Symmetricality

Perhaps one of the most common assumptions is that central incisors are perfectly symmetrical. Actually, most are not. Although the central incisors usually satisfy one of the three basic tooth forms, they are usually asymmetrical. Even in mouths where they seem to be symmetrical, close observation will usually prove otherwise.

When restoring either or both incisors, therefore, it is unnecessary to establish perfect symmetry. In fact, perfect symmetry, in some cases, could make a restoration more recognizable.

Length

Length of central incisors can vary from being only a fraction of a millimeter different to being noticeably different. Such difference can be caused by supraeruption brought about by irregular centric stops or some degree of malocclusion. It is not necessary, therefore, that a restored maxillary central incisor be the same length as its counterpart. The restoration should comply with proper occlusion, establishing centric stops, even though it might result in length differences.

Color Concentration and Location

It is common to find various degrees of color concentration in different locations of each maxillary central incisor while maintaining basic family color. Once the family color has been developed, the restoration can proceed. The color can be diluted and positioned to harmonize with the remaining dentition.

Irregularities

Irregularities are found in many teeth. Often, their location differs between the two central incisors, and irregularities are not necessarily found in both. When restoring one or both incisors, irregularities can be incorporated with little regard for exact location

Incisal Edge Position and Contour

The mandibular anterior teeth influence greatly the incisal position and contour of the maxillary central incisors. Lateral excursions and protrusive movements dictate this, hence, it is common to find differences in this area. A crowded maxillary arch, tongue thrust, and lip pressure also help position the incisal edges.

The incisal edge position and contour of a restored maxillary central incisor, therefore, should comply with the functional needs of the patient. For this reason, you should not rely entirely on the incisal edge position and contour of the unrestored central incisor; it it not necessary that they both resemble each other in this respect.

Interproximal Color

Most teeth appear to have some amount of interproximal color. Maxillary central incisors are no exception. Color reflection through the enamel is the chief source. The intensity of color varies and is influenced by shadows created by proximal tooth contour and enamel thickness.

For this reason, there should be a hint of interproximal color incorporated into almost all anterior restorations. It not only satisfies the requirements for duplicating natural dentition, it also gives the ceramist an opportunity to very subtly frame the restoration. This is especially beneficial in a multiple-unit splint; interproximal color will help make each unit appear to be individual.

Texture and Glaze

The amount of tooth texture and glaze is not the same in every mouth. When texture is present, it is usually more pronounced in the anterior area and could vary from tooth to tooth; however, both maxillary central incisors usually contain the same degree of texture and glaze; age and wear will determine this. Unlike some other characteristics, a restored maxillary central incisor should manifest the identical texture and glaze as the unrestored one.

Super Stain/Super Glaze

It has been pointed out how important it is to establish the proper degree of texture and glaze. This holds true not only for the maxillary central incisors but for any restoration seated in the mouth. While texture is mechanical and can be developed during porcelain application and/or after firing, glazing accuracy is more difficult to obtain and could be quite unpredictable. For this reason, some technicians prefer to establish glaze by applying it to the surface in the form of a liquid before final firing. Most surface or superglazes mature at temperatures lower than those necessary for body porcelains, and upon firing they mature as a thin layer of highly glazed glass. The results are unsatisfactory for several reasons, the most being the fact that the resulting glaze layer is usually microscopically porous and could eventually cause tissue damage.

Along with superglaze, superstain is often applied to the surface of the restoration to obtain needed color. The use of superstain is also undesirable. For the following reasons, superstain and superglaze should be eliminated from all ceramic restorations.

Translucency

A prime ingredient in every restoration is translucency. We must use every available means to incorporate this into a restoration. Using proper materials and techniques will help produce needed translucency. Superstain placed onto the surface of a restoration will reduce this needed translucency from 50% to 75%, depending on the type of color oxides present in the stain and the application thickness. Even though the stain might improve the color slightly, reducing the translucency is too great a price to pay.

Specular Light Reflection

Just as translucency is important to a lifelike restoration, is diffused light reflection with the absence of specular light reflection. A layer of superstain and superglaze will not permit light to enter the restoration and return in a diffused fashion. Rather, such a layer promotes specular light reflection, where the light bounces off the surface and returns to the eye, displaying little vitality.

Metamerism

Patients often complain that their restoration looks different under different light sources. This phenomenon, called *metamerism* is greatly increased when superstains are involved. The deeper that light is permitted to enter into the restoration, the less the effect metamerism will have. Internal light diffusion will tend to display the same color and lifelike qualities even in different light environments.

Underlying Colors

Superstain, when placed over porcelain colors and body modifiers, combines with these underlying colors and often produces unwanted resultant colors that violate the family color rule and usually do not harmonize with the remaining unrestored dentition.

Mouth Acids and Brushing

Even if the superstains and glazes accomplished what the technicians thought would be an improvement in the restoration, in a matter of months mouth acids and brushing can completely remove both, leaving a rough, unglazed surface that is vulnerable to discoloration and could become a source of tissue irritation and deterioration. Once this has occurred, of course, the surface cannot be recolored or reglazed.

The alternative to superstain and superglaze is internal coloration and natural glaze. The color and glaze will last the life of the restoration. Anything less is a compromise and should be eliminated from laboratory procedure.

Conclusion

The esthetics of a dental restoration is evaluated in terms of contour and color. Of the two, contour is probably the easiest to obtain or correct because it is tangible. Tooth color, however, is more difficult to obtain; it is intangible. To duplicate CTC, a thorough understanding of tooth color theory, along with its detection and measurement, is necessary. This is a team effort, made up of the person detecting and measuring the tooth color dimensions and the person duplicating these dimensions in a restoration.

Chapter 4

Irregularities in Natural Dentition

It should now be well understood that the three prerequisites for a successful restoration, whether it be a single unit or a full mandibular and maxillary case, are: (1) precise function, (2) proper contour, and (3) accurate color duplication. Function is of prime concern, often dictating contour and, occasionally, color. Only after function and contour requirements have been met is color considered. As discussed in chapter 3, the first step in duplicating tooth color is to establish a system for detecting and measuring the four tooth color dimensions: hue, chroma, maverick, and value. The direct product of the four color dimensions is *composite tooth color* (CTC). This chapter picks up at the point where CTC has already been established and describes further steps that must be taken to duplicate any specific *irregularities* that may be present in the natural dentition.

Almost all dentitions, even the most attractive and healthy, have some sot of "irregularity." These irregularities appear in the form of both contour and color and can be located internally and externally. Histologic and physiologic factors play an important role in cause, location, and extent.

External Discoloration (Fig 4-1)

Most external discolorations are merely color formations that result from food and beverage deposits coupled with poor oral hygiene. These discolorations adhere directly to the tooth surface.

Such external discoloration can be removed by scaling in conjunction with proper oral hygiene. If these deposits occur over areas of unhealthy or worn enamel, the task of removal becomes more difficult and, in some cases, impossible. If the enamel surface is etched or abnormally rough, total removal is difficult, and where the enamel is worn, such as at the incisal edge or eroded gingival area, these discolorations cannot be removed but tend to penetrate deep into the spongelike dentin, resulting in a permanent discoloration. Only after thorough scaling and pumicing can a complete color evaluation be made; any remaining color irregularity must be duplicated if one or several teeth are to be restored. This is to ensure esthetic harmony.

Internal Discoloration (Figs 4-2 to 4-4)

Internal discoloration differs substantially from external discoloration, both visually and in general oral health. All internal color found in the dentin but not responsible for the dentin color (hue-chroma) can be classified as maverick color, one of the four color dimensions that make up the tooth's composite tooth color (CTC; see chapter 3). These colors combine with the hue-chroma dimension and project their influence through the enamel, which in turn regulates their brightness. It is interesting to note that this internal discoloration, regardless how intense or unsightly, gives

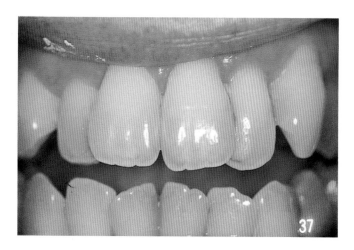

Fig 4-1 External discoloration is often the result of poor oral hygiene. Heavily textured enamel and irregular tooth alignment make it difficult to remove these color deposits. In areas of thin or deformed enamel, these colors can penetrate into the dentin, causing permanent discoloration. Exposed dentin due to worn incisal edges is especially vulnerable to discoloration; external discoloration becomes internal and impossible to control or eliminate. Color deposits found on the tooth's surface tend to be dull and lifeless and contribute nothing to true composite tooth color.

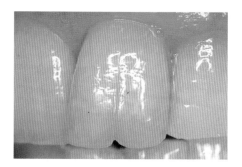

Fig 4-2

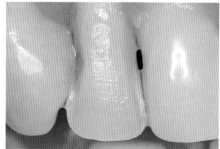

Fig 4-3

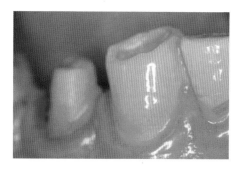

Fig 4-4

Fig 4-2 Internal tooth color found in the dentin (maverick color) contributes to CTC; it combines with dentin color and projects through the enamel as true tooth color. A clean tooth surface, free from color deposits, permits light to enter through the enamel and reflect these colors back with lifelike qualities as opposed to the dull, lifeless appearance derived from a tooth surface with unnatural color deposits.

Fig 4-3 Partially removed enamel reveals subtle maverick color dispersed throughout the dentin. In comparing the semiprepared lateral incisor with the unprepared central incisor, note the influence enamel has on CTC and also that these colors are found beneath the enamel layer, not on its surface.

Fig 4-4 When enamel is worn away, especially at the incisal edge of maxillary and mandibular anterior teeth, and dentin is exposed, tooth color change occurs rapidly. The spongelike dentin absorbs external color, which combines with the natural internal color to noticeably change the CTC. The prepared premolar indicates that the dentin has darkened to the point where fit is completely out of the normal dentin color range.

little or no indication as to the general health of the tooth. However, a high concentration of external color could indicate poor oral hygiene and unhealthy teeth and supporting periodontal tissue.

Internal color usually contributes depth and vitality to the CTC, revealing richness and dimension, whereas external discoloration displays dullness and lifelessness, blocking out potential penetrating light that could otherwise enhance CTC.

Obviously, internal color, whether it be classified as an irregularity or not, must be considered an integral component of CTC and cannot be overlooked or eliminated. External color irregularities, on the other hand, should be removed before tooth color dimensions are detected and measured.

Case Planning

Before a restorative case is started, the dentist and patient must decide which approach will be taken. Should cosmetics or conservative dentistry take priority? That is, should six maxillary anterior teeth be completely restored with full-coverage metal ceramic restorations simply because these specific irregularities have made the teeth unattractive? Or should only minor local improvements be made with minimal tooth reduction? It is important that the patient be informed of all the possibilities available and the advantages and disadvantages that are associated with each. The extent of tooth breakdown and the limited amount that can be tolerated by the patient must be left to the judgment of the dentist with full confidence that whichever choice is made, whether it be to restore multiple teeth for the sake of cosmetics or a single tooth for the sake of conservation, the laboratory can comply with these esthetic demands.

Perhaps the simplest solution to many cases is to restore multiple units, making changes that improve esthetics throughout the entire mouth. In most cases, however, the laboratory is called on to duplicate color and irregularities associated with single units. To ensure an exact duplication, all pertinent information must be presented to the laboratory. Before irregularities can be considered, the four color dimensions must be detected and measured. Upon completing this, irregularities are located and defined; with little exception, most can be categorized as to location: (1) root and gingival third, (2) middle third, (3) incisal third, and (4) entire labial surface (Fig 4-5).

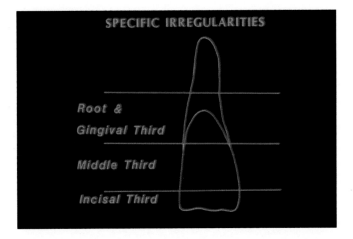

Fig 4-5 In order for the laboratory to successfully duplicate color irregularities, the technician and dentist should both have some idea as to where these irregularities are located and how they can be identified. Although there cannot be an absolute rule for location, most irregularities are common to certain areas of the tooth. The tooth can be divided into thirds, and in most cases location is predictable. Along with the entire labial surface, irregularities can be located predominantly in the root and gingival, middle, and incisal thirds of the tooth. During color dimension detection and measurement, these four locations should be thoroughly scrutinized.

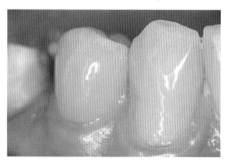

Fig 4-6

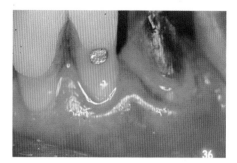

Fig 4-7

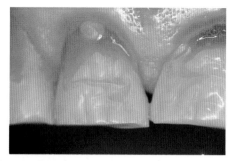

Fig 4-8

Fig 4-6   Erosion is gradual and may go unnoticed until sensitivity and/or discoloration occurs. The mandibular right canine and first premolar in this case show first signs of gingival erosion. Improper oral hygiene, thin enamel at the gingival third of the tooth, and tissue resorption can initiate erosion in this area.

Fig 4-7   With further tissue resorption and enamel wear, erosion becomes more pronounced. Dentin and root structure become more exposed, promoting drastic change to composite tooth color. With this amount of exposure, the entire dentin will eventually become discolored through absorption and chemical change; the prepared tooth indicates this and also that the restoration must include not only the needed dentin color to match the remaining dentition but also the eroded contour.

Fig 4-8   Advanced gingival erosion coupled with enamel deterioration exposes labial dentin. Ideally, the entire segment should be restored. However, occasionally, only one tooth in the midst of several other broken-down teeth requires immediate attention. In cases such as this, erosion and color must be duplicated exactly so as to maintain harmony with the remaining dentition. This is a good example of dentin discoloration that is completely out of natural tooth color range. Color dimension detection and measurement would be simple using the maverick customized tooth color guide.

Irregularities in the Root and Gingival Third (Figs 4-6 to 4-8)

Out of all the areas of the tooth, the root and gingival third will exhibit the most irregularities. In this area, enamel is thin and vulnerable to wear. Even under healthy conditions, this thin enamel layer permits more dentin color to show through than any other part of the tooth. This color intensifies with the slightest wearing away of the enamel. Here, the enamel can become thin enough to permit discoloration from certain foods and beverages to actually penetrate through the enamel rods and cause the underlying soft dentin to become color saturated. With more severe wear and gingival resorption, erosion will occur in both the root and gingival third of the tooth crown. As gingival resorption and tooth wear worsen, erosion and discoloration become more pronounced and can indeed be classified as irregularities that must be duplicated if any of the teeth in that vicinity are to be restored. Teeth in this condition can survive for many years in an otherwise healthy state and may not ever require treatment throughout the life of the patient; however, if for some reason, one or several need treatment in the form of a restoration, it is essential to duplicate both the erosion (contour) and discoloration.

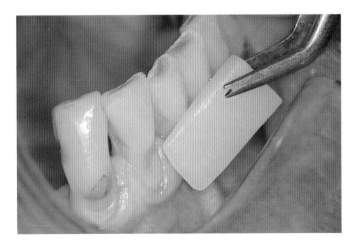

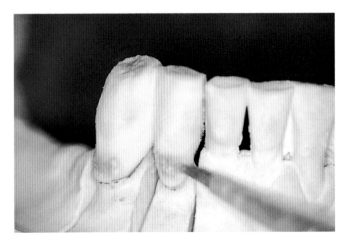

Fig 4-9a Mandibular right canine and lateral incisor are being restored for functional reasons. Erosion in the gingival third of the teeth produces discoloration that must be duplicated in the restorations so that color harmony can be maintained with the remaining dentition. During tooth preparation, the mid and incisal third of these teeth were found to retain normal dentin color (hue-chroma dimension), and it was decided to use two methods for duplicating these color dimensions: embedded maverick and deep-stain maverick.

Fig 4-9b Embedded maverick and deep-stain maverick methods for color dimension duplication were combined in this instance because both have several features in common. The dentin color is in the normal tooth color range and color concentration exists in several locations (gingival third and incisal edge). After complete body buildup (hue-chroma), these areas are scooped out and replaced with body modifiers and stain (maverick color). After proper condensing and shaping, the porcelain is fired.

Color Detection, Measurement, and Duplication

The first step in restoration is to semiprepare the tooth to determine how much influence discoloration has on the CTC. In removing half of the enamel just to the dentinoenamel junction, it not only enables detection and measurement of the tooth color dimensions, it also shows the effect the color irregularity has and the most appropriate method for duplicating the entire CTC.

Once half the enamel surface is removed, either one of two color involvements will be evident: (1) the color influence will be localized and affect only the root and gingival third of the tooth crown, leaving the hue-chroma as a separate color dimension; or (2) the color influence will affect the entire dentin to the point where the dentin is totally saturated with maverick color, taking it completely out of the color range of the hue-chroma color

guide. In this situation, the maverick dimension becomes the hue-chroma, which means that only two color dimensions are involved in the composite color of this tooth: maverick and value (enamel).

After you have detected and measured the color dimensions, the next step is to decide which of the duplicating methods is most appropriate for the restoration.

Case 1—Hue-Chroma, Maverick, and Value (Figs 4-9a to d)

If semi-preparation of the tooth reveals that the discoloration is localized in the root and gingival third of the tooth, with no effect on the mid and incisal third, there are two duplicating methods to

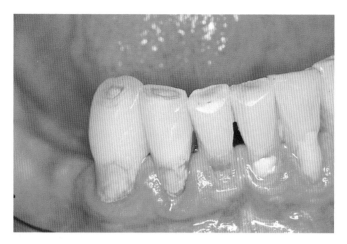

Fig 4-9c After firing, the restoration is contoured and glazed. Although the prime reason for restoring these teeth was functional (to recontour the incisal edges so as to take on more load responsibility with a removable partial denture during lateral excursion), the esthetic aspect was also considered; had the erosion and discoloration at the gingival third been ignored, disharmony with the remaining dentition would have been obvious.

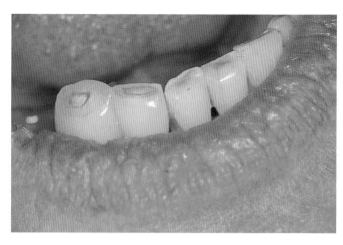

Fig 4-9d The body modifiers and stain for the incisal edge were selected, using the colors found in the incisal edges of the remaining dentition. Often these color concentrations vary from tooth to tooth, but the family color is usually the same. Even though function is more important, esthetic harmony should not be overlooked.

choose from: (1) embedded maverick, and (2) deep stain maverick.

1. *Embedded maverick.* The embedded maverick method for duplication is accomplished by embedding the detected maverick color in the exact location it was found in the prepared tooth. The colors are applied after the initial body (dentin) buildup.
   a. *Opaque.* The opaque is applied in two separate firings. The first consists of a thin opaque wash. The selection is dictated by the hue-chroma dimension for the restoration. The opaque is mixed with an opaque medium or distilled water. This is fired to full maturing temperature for opaque. The transition layer consists of approximately one third each of opaque, dentin porcelain, and body modifier. The maturing temperature for this layer must be 10° to 15°F lower than the original temperature.

   b. *Dentin build-up.* The dentin porcelain is applied, leaving enough space for full coverage of enamel porcelain. Dentin porcelain in the root and gingival third is removed to make room for the selected maverick color. The maverick selection should match the irregularity in this area in both color and contour. The entire restoration is covered with enamel porcelain and fired. After final contouring and surface texturing, the restoration is glazed and made ready for seating.

2. *Deep stain maverick.* Although the deep stain maverick is primarily used for thin restorations where there is too little room for embedding modifiers, it works well in cases where certain accent colors of high concentration are required to satisfy the duplication of irregularities. In many situations, stains are preferred over modifiers because of their potency and the fact that their effectiveness can be con-

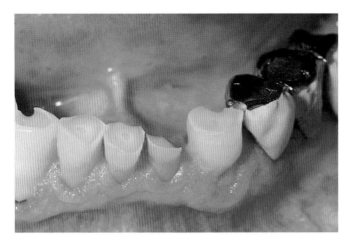

Fig 4-10a Severely worn teeth coupled with deteriorating posterior restorations. It was decided to restore the fractured left lateral incisor, with intentions to restore the entire arch at a later date. In cases such as this where the entire dentin has discolored into the maverick color range, the maverick and enamel duplicating method is obviously most appropriate; the dentin color is completely out of the hue-chroma color range. Therefore, just two color dimensions are of concern: maverick and value.

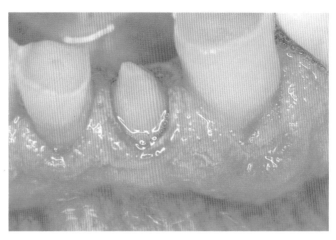

Fig 4-10b Prepared mandibular left lateral incisor ready for impressions. Eroded gingival third of the tooth made it impossible to prepare a shoulder for a porcelain margin. In order to comply with the eroded areas found on the central incisor and canine, the casting must be feather edged in this area so color can be obtained in a very thin layer of porcelain.

trolled simply by diluting them with liquid medium. The stains can be used alone or in conjunction with modifiers; after establishing a basic family color with a modifier, stains may be embedded in certain areas for effect. This is called "color on color" and is very effective when the root and gingival third exhibit color irregularities. This area is built up with body modifiers. Then with the help of stain, certain highlights and accents are established, using adjacent natural teeth to dictate color, concentration, and location.

In cases where the hue-chroma dimension is obvious and the only irregularity is located in the root and eroded gingival third area, the dentin buildup is carried out to full contour in the same manner as usual. The eroded area is shaped to conform with the surrounding teeth, and in lieu of body modifiers, all the discoloration is achieved

by incorporating stain into the raw porcelain. The stain should be mixed with stain medium rather than distilled water. Liquid medium tends to hold the color oxides together better than water, but care must be taken to make certain the porcelain is in a semiwet state so it will not pull the liquid from the stain mixture. Also, the stain mixture must be mixed well into the porcelain, using slight vibration so as to permit the glycerine content of the medium to mix with the buildup liquid in the porcelain. After thorough drying, the restoration is fired, contoured, and glazed.

Case 2—Maverick and Enamel (Figs 4-10a to i)

If semipreparation of the tooth reveals that eroded discoloration extends throughout the entire dentin, usually the dentin color is out of the hue-chroma

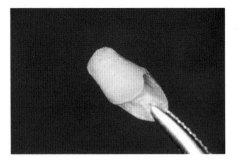

Fig 4-10c

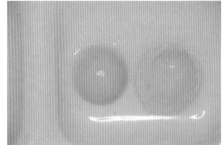

Fig 4-10d

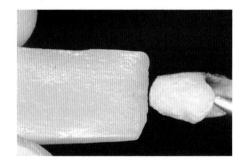

Fig 4-10e

Fig 4-10c   The opaque layer is a thin wash of prescribed opaque for the selected maverick color (opaque from any porcelain system can be used, but for more accurate results a customized maverick color system is recommended). The opaque should block out approximately 50% of the underlying color. Note gray substructure slightly showing through the opaque wash.

Fig 4-10d   When a standard porcelain kit is used, the transition layer must be mixed (half prescribed opaque and half body modifier). The combination is mixed well and applied over the fired opaque wash, establishing a rough surface. When using the Maverick Porcelain System kit, the transition layer is premixed for each maverick selection, making it possible to obtain a more accurate result.

Fig 4-10e   The fired transition layer is compared to the selected customized color tab. The purpose of this layer is to (1) block out the remaining 50% color influence and (2) resemble as close as possible the maverick color dimension selected for the restoration. Note rough surface for diffusing light entering the restoration.

customized color range. This also shows that the only two color dimensions to be concerned with in this case are maverick and value, and that the most logical method of duplication would be maverick and enamel.

After selecting the proper maverick (dentin) and incisal (enamel) from the respective CTC guides, the next step is to decide on the most appropriate opaque. The basic color family must be determined. Using the Vita Lumin system as a basis, we can categorize the oranges and browns as being in the "A" series, the yellows in the "B" series, and gray in the "C" series. The selected maverick color is also categorized and the darkest opaque in that particular family is used for the restoration (ie, light brown, dark brown, and orange fall in the "A" family, whereas yellow and honey yellow

would be considered "B" family A4 and B4 opaque, respectively).

1. *Opaque.* In the maverick and enamel method for duplication, the opaque wash is either A4 or B4, depending on the maverick selection. The transition layer consists of one half opaque and one half maverick color.
2. *Dentin buildup.* In the maverick and enamel method, the entire dentin buildup is comprised of maverick (body modifier) plus the portion of neutral porcelain required for desaturation. This is built to a contour that leaves enough room for enamel porcelain to completely cover the restoration. It can be fired alone or with a separate enamel firing, or they can be combined in a single firing. Separate firings allow

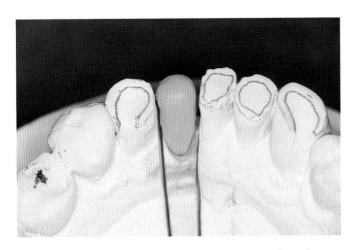

Fig 4-10f Fired maverick body buildup is placed onto the master working model and evaluated, making sure no functional problem exists and that there is sufficient room available for enamel porcelain. An advantage in firing the enamel porcelain separately is that it gives the ceramist an opportunity to adjust the dentin if more room is needed. However, both dentin and enamel can be applied and fired together.

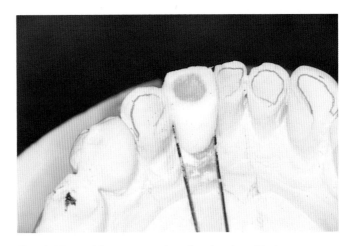

Fig 4-10g After comparing the dentin with the customized shade tab and finding the color to be correct, the enamel porcelain is applied. It is advisable, when possible, to draw a dentinoenamel junction on the worn incisal edges of the anterior teeth of the master working model; this gives the ceramist a guide to follow as to the needed thickness and contour of the applied enamel porcelain. Note that the enamel covers the surrounding teeth.

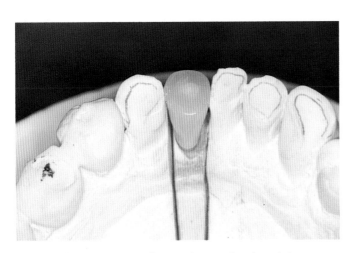

Fig 4-10h The enamel porcelain is fired and the restoration is placed onto the master working model and reevaluated. If care was taken during enamel porcelain application, only minor adjustment will be necessary, after which the restoration is refined and glazed. The restoration is now ready to be seated.

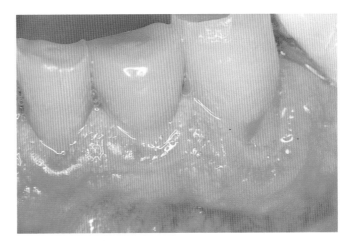

Fig 4-10i Seated left lateral restoration. The color and contour of the gingival third blends well with surrounding dentition with no sign of opaque or metal margin. In areas such as this (approximately 0.2 mm), the transition layer plays a major role in that it contains all the color needed for the CTC. Additional body modifiers and stains can be incorporated into this area as well as into the dentin layer to ensure perfect color harmony. The results show how appropriate the maverick and enamel method of duplication was for this restoration.

for color evaluation and could prevent a need for alterations. A comparison with a customized tab can be made after the initial firing before the enamel firing.

After contouring, paying special attention to the gingival erosion, the restoration is glazed.

The root and gingival third of the tooth play important roles in overall contour and color. They are areas often overlooked when duplicating CTC. Most teeth that have deteriorated to the point where a restoration is necessary exhibit some degree of gingival involvement, ranging from minor resorption to major tissue damage with erosion and discoloration. Care must be taken to duplicate this area precisely. A restoration that does not include this information stands out as unnatural and may be unacceptable to the patient.

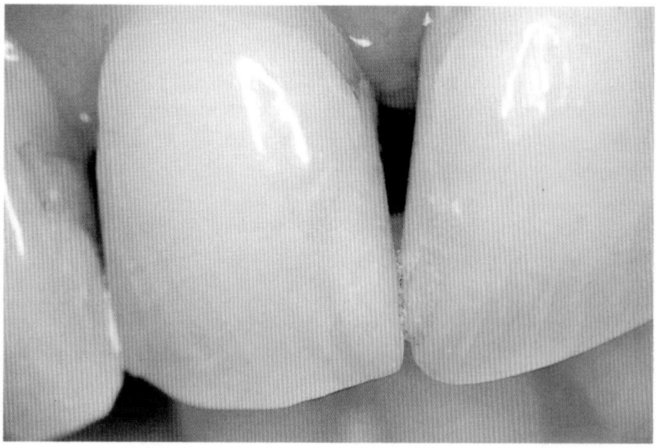

Fig 4-11 Interproximal restorations are a common irregularity found in the middle third of the tooth. They are prone to discoloration because of the chemical makeup of the material and the difficulty in performing proper oral hygiene due to location. If a restoration is to be placed next to or in the vicinity of an interproximal restoration, in some cases it is advisable to include one in porcelain.

Irregularities in the Middle Third

Most irregularities in the middle third are confined to the interproximal areas in the form of restorations and natural color deposits.

Interproximal Restorations

Almost every interproximal restoration will eventually discolor. If the restoration is next to or in the vicinity of a discolored restoration, it might be necessary to incorporate this discoloration so that esthetic harmony can be maintained (Fig 4-11). This should be discussed during case planning so the patient can decide.

This irregularity usually consists of the discolored restoration surrounded by a thin seepage line that is of a more concentrated color, and it is usually incorporated after the porcelain is built up to full contour. The area is scooped out and the walls are refined with a sharp instrument to give it added depth. The wall is then coated with a very

thin covering of stain while the porcelain is still in a semiwet state. The porcelain must not be dry enough to pull the liquid from the stain nor wet enough to permit the stain to spread. The scooped out area is embedded with modifiers selected from the customized maverick shade tab that matches the discolored filling material. Even though the filled area of the tooth is not covered with enamel, it is advisable to cover the restored irregularity with enamel porcelain along with the rest of the restoration. This provides color depth and authenticity. It is followed by contouring and glaze (Figs 4-12a to c).

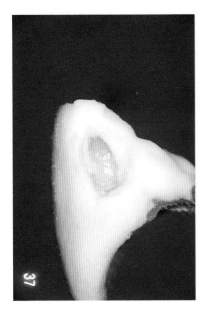

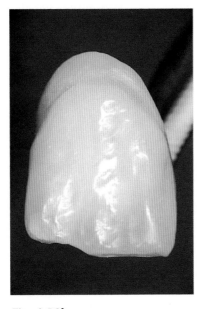

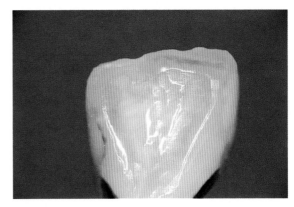

Fig 4-12a

Fig 4-12b

Fig 4-12c

Fig 4-12a Interproximal area of built-up crown is scooped out and contoured to desired size and shape. The walls of the scooped-out areas are stained and the cavity is filled with a selected modifier. Color intensity can vary from subtle to intensive, depending on needed results. The restoration is then covered with a thin layer of enamel porcelain and fired.

Fig 4-12b Labial surface of maxillary right central incisor restoration with subtle interproximal restoration (mesial). A distal restoration with more intense color is almost unnoticeable labially because of its lingual location.

Fig 4-12c Lingual view of same crown as in Fig 4-12b, comparing subtle mesial restoration with the more pronounced distal restoration placed lingually to complement the surrounding dentition.

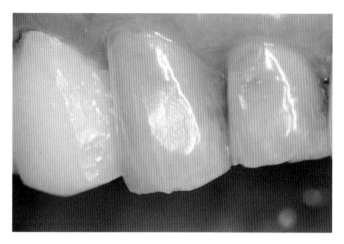

Fig 4-13 Maxillary right canine displays a high concentration of interproximal color. When compared to the provisional restoration on the first premolar, it is obvious that for the final restoration to be acceptable it must include this interproximal color (along with other irregularities that will be discussed later). Although these colors may be extremely concentrated in the surrounding dentition, the restoration could contain a less concentrated version, while maintaining the same color family, and still be acceptable.

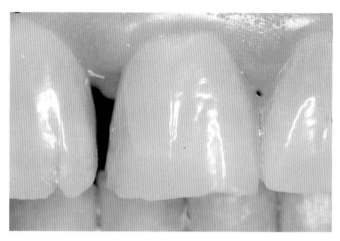

Fig 4-14 Maxillary left central incisor with very subtle interproximal color. This can be found in most teeth and therefore should be included in most restorations. This is especially appropriate in connected multiunit restorations; the subtle interproximal color will help make each unit appear separate, thus adding to the esthetic value.

Interproximal Coloration (Figs 4-13 and 4-14)

Most natural dentition has some degree of interproximal discoloration, and any restoration to be seated in the vicinity of interproximal discoloration must contain this color irregularity, duplicating family color, concentration, and location.

The colors are duplicated by embedding body modifiers in these areas during dentin buildup or by using stains that correspond to the detected color. Duplication differs somewhat from that of interproximal restorations in that a demarcation stain is not included; there is no seepage involved.

Even though interproximal color is usually limited to the surface, some color will penetrate the enamel, making it impossible to remove. These colors vary from a diluted yellow-orange to light and dark brown, depending on the patient's eating and drinking habits. Tea, coffee, tobacco, and certain medications are common sources of interproximal discoloration. The degree of oral hygiene will have some influence on the extent of this condition, but it is almost impossible to eliminate it completely.

Irregularities in the middle third are limited to interproximal restoration discolorations and color deposits that may be very subtle, yet to eliminate these subtleties from a restoration could mean a mediocre final product, as opposed to possible perfection.

Irregularities in the Incisal and Occlusal Third

Perhaps the most influential portion of the tooth associated with function and esthetic harmony is the incisal and buccal third. Incisal position and contour of the six maxillary anterior teeth are the major contributors to proper phonetics and function. While the lingual aspect is directly responsible for anterior guidance and speech, the labial third position is responsible for lip support, and its incisal edge contour promotes biting and function. The importance of the incisal third, therefore, must not be overlooked. The degree of success in any restoration depends greatly on how much attention is placed in this area.

Obtaining optimum results does not end with acceptable function and contour, however. Effort must be made to capture every visible landmark found on teeth adjacent to the restoration in this area. Some of the irregularities found here are common only to the incisal and buccal third, whereas others can, on occasion, be found in other areas of the tooth.

Incisal Frame

The incisal edge of the maxillary and mandibular six anterior teeth generally shows little or no demarcation between dentin and enamel. Many teeth exhibit what seems to be no enamel at all, just dense, nontranslucent dentin, even though enamel is indeed present (Fig 4-15).

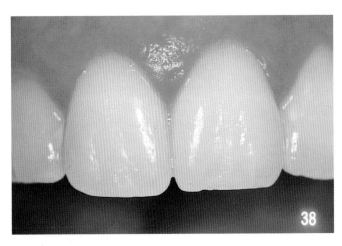

Fig 4-15 Maxillary central incisors with subtle incisal enamel; gradual transition from the middle to the incisal third makes it difficult to recognize in many teeth. Some teeth, however, have a distinct enamel band extending interproximally.

Some teeth do, however, possess a thin band of enamel that frames the incisal edge and in many cases extends interproximally to its middle third. The frame has a halo effect and can range from translucency to transparency, depending on incisal wear and enamel thickness in this area. Its band width can measure from a fraction to 1.5 mm and is usually of uniform width. When duplicating this, care must be taken during porcelain buildup to incorporate the exact dimensions.

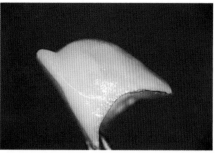

Fig 4-16a 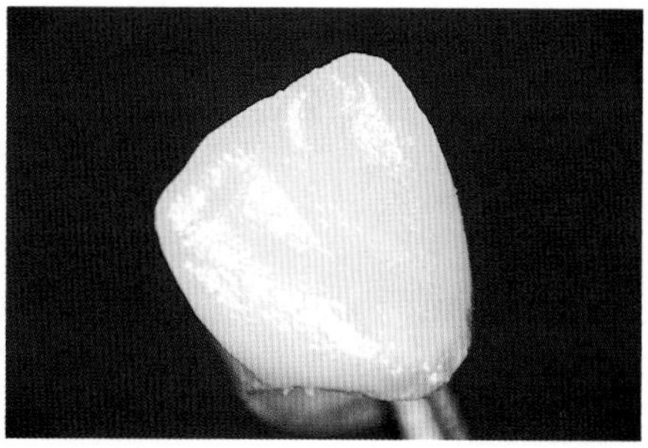   **Fig 4-16b**

Fig 4-16a   To ensure exact enamel location the restoration can be "shell fired." The enamel and needed color are fired over the transition layer in exact locations.

Fig 4-16b   Lingual view of shell-fired restoration. At this stage, the restoration is placed back onto the master working model and is contoured to the exact length according to functional needs. Once this has been accomplished with exact incisal edge contour and position, other required irregularities can be incorporated into the incisal third of the restoration with the assurance they will not be eliminated during final contouring.

Shell Fire (Figs 4-16a and b)

To ensure exact location of the duplicated irregularity in the restoration, a process called "shell firing" can be used. Shell firing simply involves a shell fired over the transition layer and is designed to outline the exact outer dimensions of the restoration. After firing, the shell is placed back onto the working model and contoured to proper functional length and width. Once the desired dimensions have been established, it can be safely assumed that what is left will not be removed during final shaping and glazing. Also, anything added to the shell within these confines will remain with no concern that it will be ground away.

The incisal frame can be included during the shell buildup. If its width and length are satisfactory upon shell completion, the remainder of the restoration can be built to full contour, then final contour and glaze. If the desired results are not obtained during shell firing, adjustments can be made before the fabrication is completed. Proper incisal porcelain must be selected to give the correct amount of translucency or transparency that coincides with the adjacent natural dentition. To misjudge or eliminate this does not necessarily indicate failure, but including it enhances the restoration.

Dentin Frame

The dentin frame resembles the incisal frame in that it also borders the incisal edge. The main difference is that it is not translucent or transparent but is opaque. In many cases it is the same or

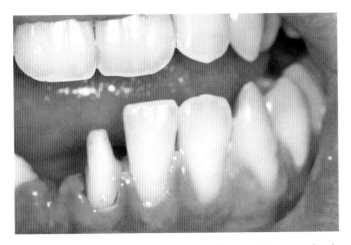

Fig 4-17 "Dentin frame" especially prominent on both maxillary central incisors. It is referred to as dentin frame because it resembles dentin color of the tooth. Even though in a natural dentition the frame may be caused by color reflected through the enamel, in the restoration it must be included by placing dentin porcelain into the incisal edge; porcelain does not reflect color in the same manner as dental enamel.

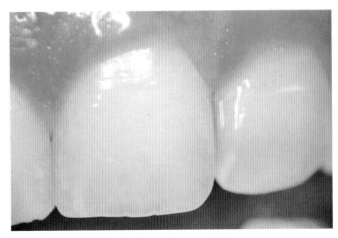

Fig 4-18 Maxillary left central incisor with "maverick frame." The maverick dimension, which contributes to the composite color of the tooth, is quite obvious; it is dispersed throughout the incisal third. As in the case with a dentin frame, the maverick frame is usually derived from a reflection. To duplicate this, modifiers and/or stains are used.

very close to the hue-chroma of the tooth, thus its name, "dentin frame" (Fig 4-17).

The dentin frame can be incorporated into the restoration using much the same procedure as with the incisal frame. Shell firing is used, carrying it to full length and width while building the dentin and enamel porcelain into their proper location. The length and interproximal areas are trimmed back to allow for the thin band of dentin that will complete its length and width. The dentin (hue-chroma) selected for the restoration is used as the framing material. Dentin framing is found more often on the maxillary central incisors than on the mandibular incisors. After completing the addition to the shell, the buildup is completed, fired, contoured, and glazed.

Maverick Frame

The only difference between dentin and maverick frame is the basic color. While the dentin frame is the actual hue-chroma dimension of the tooth, the maverick frame is made up of the maverick dimension found in the tooth. The intensity of the maverick frame may vary from tooth to tooth but the basic family color usually prevails (Fig 4-18).

As in the case of the incisal and dentin frame, the most accurate way to duplicate the maverick frame is with the shell firing technique. One difference is that the maverick color in this area can be duplicated with either body modifier or stain. Modifiers can be incorporated during porcelain buildup over the fired shell. After complete porce-

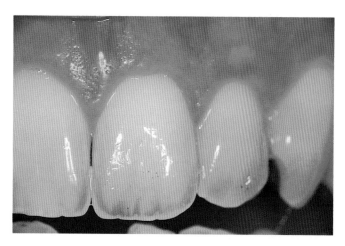

Fig 4-19 Maxillary anterior teeth with transparency in the incisal third. Most teeth have no transparency, but for teeth that do, it is usually found in the incisal third and in many cases is caused by a thin incisal edge, brought about by wear.

lain buildup, stain is applied in the desired area. The stain is first mixed with liquid stain medium to keep color particles together. When brushing stain into semiwet porcelain, vibrate it slightly with a serrated instrument to ensure complete color absorption. Care must be taken to vibrate it sufficiently so as to mix the liquid medium in the stain with the liquid in the porcelain buildup. The porcelain buildup should be such that only minor contouring is necessary after firing. The restoration is then glazed and ready for placement.

Transparent Incisal

A transparent object is one that permits light to pass through it freely with no diffusion (eg, clear glass). A translucent object, on the other hand, does not permit light to pass through it freely (eg, frosted glass). Most teeth have no transparency. Therefore, as a general rule, any material or

procedure used during fabrication that will lend to transparency should be avoided. It is the quality of translucency that is generally important to replicate. This is because we rely on light for transmitting color and lifelikeness (without light there would be no color), and this is accomplished through translucency, which scatters light and color in a diffused fashion. A lifelike restoration is directly proportional to the depth at which color is placed in a restoration and the amount of light diffusion. A transparent environment will not diffuse color; it simply permits light to pass through. A translucent environment, on the other hand, will permit light to enter, bounce from color particle to color particle, and return to the eye in a scattered fashion.

There are occasions, however, when transparency is indeed found in natural dentition. When duplicating the CTC of a tooth or teeth that possess transparency, this must be included in the restoration. When transparency is present, it is usually located in the incisal third of maxillary and mandibular incisors (Fig 4-19). Every porcelain kit contains transparent or clear porcelains that are used in restorations that require this. The degree of transparency dictates at what stage during porcelain buildup the transparent porcelain will be incorporated. (Total transparency seldom exists; there is usually some degree of translucency.) The higher the degree of transparency, the sooner the transparent porcelain is added with the least amount of underlying body (dentin) porcelain.

As far as substructure design is concerned, to obtain optimum results in the transparent area, metal should be eliminated (but only with the assurance that strength will not be compromised). In the event that metal support is essential, steps should be taken to block out its influence and thus permit as much transparency as possible. The degree of transparency will also dictate the foundation material and the amount of each. A very thin layer of dentin porcelain can act as the foundation, thick enough to block out the underlying opaque but thin enough to not diminish the transparency.

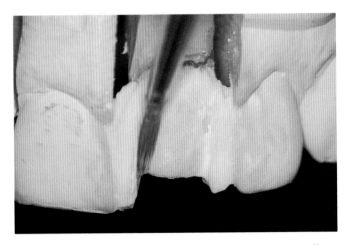

Fig 4-20a Incorporating transparency into maxillary left central incisor restoration. One of several methods is to include transparent porcelain and other needed irregularities during vertical layering of dentin.

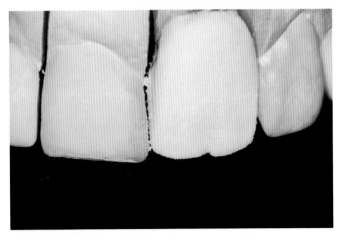

Fig 4-20b Completed dentin buildup, ready to be fired.

Transparency is built into the restoration, mimicking the tooth to be duplicated (Figs 4-20a to g). Observing the natural dentition will help the ceramist decide exactly how the transparency should be incorporated into the restoration. There are three basic methods to achieve this: (1) horizontal layering, (2) vertical layering, and (3) random deposits.

Horizontal Layering

Transparent powder is laid down evenly mesiodistally and is usually located at the incisal edge. Occasionally, this may migrate well into the incisal third, giving way to translucency with eventual opacity as it nears the middle third of the tooth's crown.

Vertical Layering

Transparent powder is applied to the restoration in the form of vertical incisogingival sections that are separated by areas of dentin. These areas of

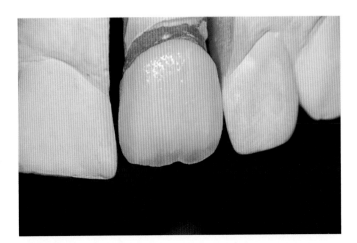

Fig 4-20c Fired dentin layer, including transparency (incisally and interproximally) and other irregularities, along with hue-chroma and maverick color dimensions needed for CTC.

transparency are built in a vertical fashion and are usually located interproximally and primarily toward the incisal third. Its effect diminishes toward the middle third of the tooth.

155

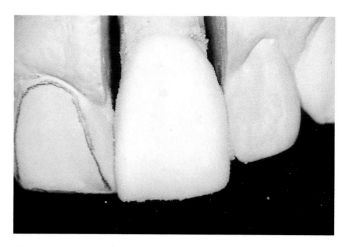

Fig 4-20d After covering dentin with enamel porcelain, areas are scooped out and filled with more transparent porcelain powder, recontoured, and overbuilt slightly to compensate for shrinkage. Enamel layer is now ready to be fired.

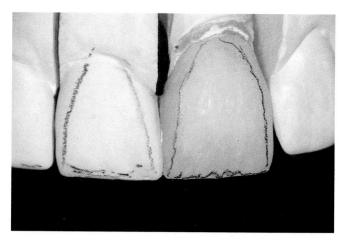

Fig 4-20e Restoration after slight contouring (using right central incisor as a guide) ready to be glazed. If careful contouring is done during enamel buildup, little contouring will be needed after firing.

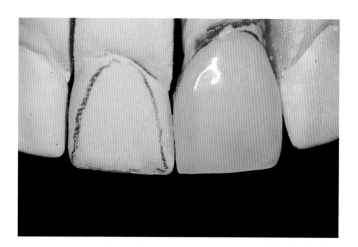

Fig 4-20f Glazed restoration on master working model ready for seating.

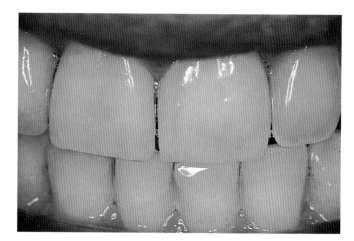

Fig 4-20g Seated maxillary left central incisor restoration showing a random transparency that harmonizes well with the remaining anterior teeth. Areas of transparency should not be placed in exact locations found in adjacent teeth. In the natural dentition, these locations vary from tooth to tooth. (Patient requested the same diastema between central incisors as existed before treatment.)

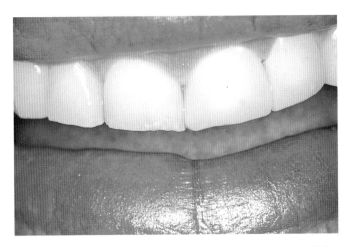

Fig 4-21a Compare the provisional restorations of the left central and lateral incisors with the right central and lateral incisors. Color improvements must be made on the permanent restorations even though the provisional restorations blend well with the surrounding dentition.

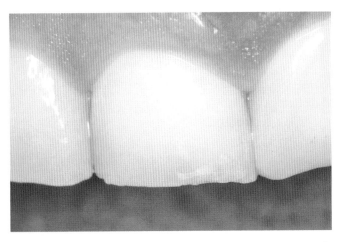

Fig 4-21b The right central incisor reveals maverick deposits that should be included in the permanent restoration of the left central incisor. Along with interproximal color and hypocalcification (to be discussed), the most obvious irregularity is maverick deposits in the incisal third. Worn incisal edge is probably the cause for discoloration in this area.

Random Deposits

Some teeth show random areas of transparency. These deposits of transparency vary in size, shape, and location and are easily reproduced by scooping out dentin porcelain after full buildup, contour, and filling these areas with transparent porcelain powder. Building the restoration to full contour before carrying out this procedure minimizes the need for excessive contouring after firing. This could help prevent the possibility of removing these transparent deposits in favor of obtaining proper contour before glaze.

Maverick Deposits (Figs 4-21a to l)

Deposits of color (maverick) are found more often than transparency in the incisal third of the anterior teeth. These color deposits are usually formed due to worn lingual and incisal edge enamel. The worn areas leave the underlying dentin unprotected and vulnerable to discoloration. The relatively spongy dentin becomes discolored when it contacts certain foods and beverages during mastication. Regardless how meticulous a person is with oral hygiene, these color irregularities seem to form with advanced age and wear.

Duplicating this condition in a restoration is simple in that body modifiers and stains can be used during porcelain buildup. When room permits, body modifiers should be used rather than stain because their effects can be better regulated. When space is a problem and the area is thin, stains will suit the purpose even though care must be taken not to overemphasize color, due to the great potency of stains. In most cases, these color areas are subtle and using the maverick buildup method of duplication usually works well because the color is covered over with a thin layer of dentin and enamel porcelain. When the restoration is to be placed next to natural dentition, it is

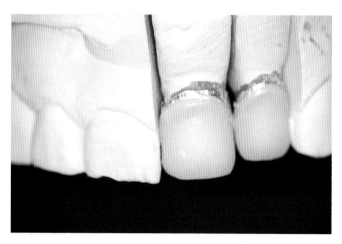

Fig 4-21c　When establishing porcelain margins (platinum foil method), maverick deposits are made over the transition layer. It is important to place these colors deep into the restoration to ensure a more lifelike result. The color family should be duplicated but in most cases should be less pronounced than that found in the surrounding dentition.

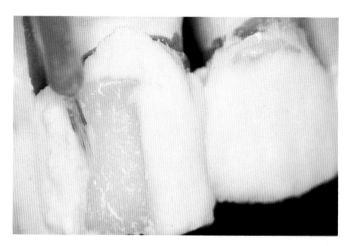

Fig 4-21d　Vertical layering of dentin, incorporating other needed irregularities and applied over previously applied maverick deposits. Body modifiers and stains are used to supply these colors.

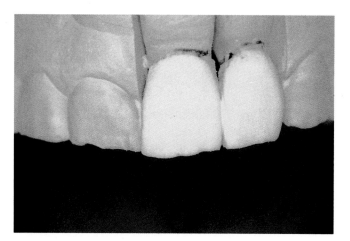

Fig 4-21e　A thin layer of enamel porcelain is applied over dentin and is overbuilt slightly to compensate for shrinkage during firing. Precise contouring at this stage is imperative; any excessive grinding after firing might remove needed irregularities and colors that were placed in the restoration to satisfy CTC.

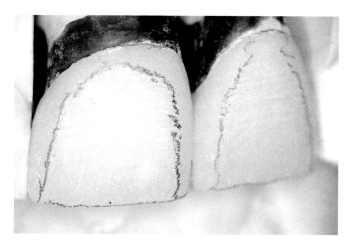

Fig 4-21f　After minor contouring, using right central and lateral incisors as guides for esthetics and the articulated mandibular model for functional requirements, the restorations are ready to be glazed (note that the platinum foil at the labial margins remains in place during glaze stage).

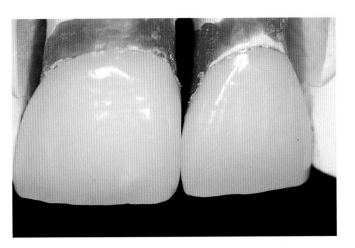

Fig 4-21g Glazed restorations ready for platinum removal from labial margins. For anterior restorations, porcelain margins should be considered whenever possible (for more information on the platinum foil method for developing porcelain margins, see chapter 2).

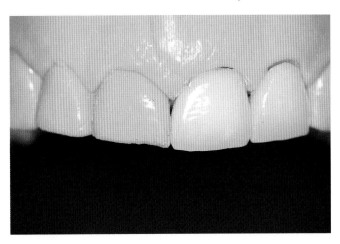

Fig 4-21h Completed restorations seated on tissue model. Even though properly located color deposits (maverick buildup) are important esthetically for this case, precise contour in the gingival area will ensure optimum tissue health. Without the aid of the tissue model, this would be impossible.

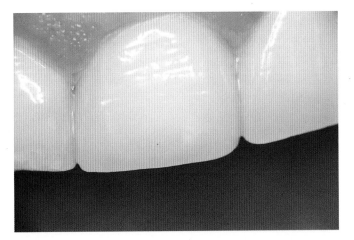

Fig 4-21i Seated restorations reveal maverick deposits in the incisal third and several other subtle irregularities (ie, enamel craze lines, hypocalcification, and interproximal color). In most cases, the patient prefers that when these irregularities are included in a restoration they be more subtle than those found in the remaining dentition. (Note how well the tissue has adapted to the well glazed porcelain margin only 3 days after seating.)

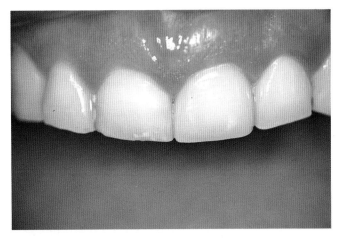

Fig 4-21j Seated maxillary left central and lateral incisors blend well with other natural anterior teeth. Tissue model (Fig 4-21h) helped ensure healthy gingivae along with a well-sealed porcelain margin.

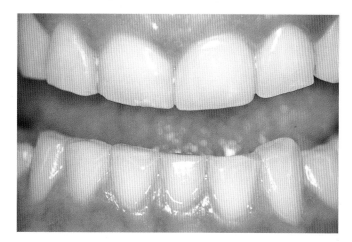

Fig 4-21k Functional aspect of seated restorations. Note worn incisal edges of mandibular anterior teeth. This was the cause of the incisal wear on the maxillary anterior teeth, which wore away the enamel and exposed the dentin that eventually discolored.

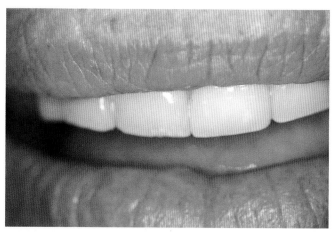

Fig 4-21l Maverick deposits in the incisal third of the left central incisor restoration blend with those located in the right central incisor, verifying the importance of incorporating these irregularities into an otherwise lifeless restoration.

advisable to underaccentuate rather than to overaccentuate this irregularity because of the effect of metamerism. The more subtle, the less pronounced under certain given lighting conditions.

Incisal Edge Maverick

This irregularity resembles "maverick deposits," the main difference being that the discoloration is found only on the biting edge. The color does not project through the enamel on the lingual or labial surfaces. Although anterior maxillary teeth are affected as well, the anterior mandibular teeth are more noticeable because of their location in the oral cavity (Fig 4-22).

Incisal edge maverick is usually attributed to enamel wear at the incisal edge of anterior teeth. As the enamel in this area wears and becomes thinner, the underlying dentin becomes more vulnerable to discoloration. Certain foods and beverages, along with tobacco and cigarettes, con-

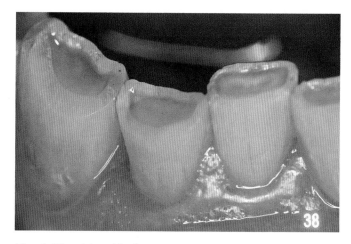

Fig 4-22 Mandibular anterior teeth showing worn enamel and exposed dentin at the incisal edge. Wear on the incisal edge of anterior teeth varies from mouth to mouth, ranging from very slight enamel abrasion where worn facets are visible in the enamel to exposed dentin that is worn almost to the pulp. When restoring an entire arch, some improvement can be made to satisfy the esthetics of the restoration. However, when just one or several are to be restored, exact duplication is essential.

tribute to this; the dentin readily absorbs and displays them in a noticeable fashion. The amount of absorption and concentration depends greatly on: (1) the amount of enamel wear, (2) eating and drinking habits of the patient, (3) use of tobacco and cigarettes, (4) how the body reacts to "foreign elements," and (5) the oral hygiene habits of the patient.

When detecting and measuring the four tooth color dimensions, it is important that this irregularity be included in the treatment plan. The involvement is restricted to the incisal edge and affects only the dentin in that area, maintaining the other color dimensions (hue-chroma and value) that make up the tooth's CTC.

When duplicating this condition in a restoration that involves less than the six anterior teeth, and especially where only one or two incisors are affected, it is important to select the exact color family and concentration. The customized maverick color guide can measure this accurately. If the restoration includes all six anterior teeth, the possibility of color change is good not only in hue, chroma, and value, but also the incisal edge discoloration. Should this alternative be considered, however, a certain amount of discoloration must be incorporated into the restoration in order to maintain esthetic harmony. Any drastic change for the sake of making the restoration "younger" could produce an unnatural result. In cases that exhibit incisal edge discoloration, some degree of wear is also evident and should be made part of the restoration.

When including incisal edge maverick, the restoration is processed using one of the eight methods used to duplicate CTC. The porcelain is built and shaped to full contour, making certain all excursions are worked into the basic functional aspect of the case. This will ensure that the exact length of the restoration is obtained before the alterations are performed. Once this is accomplished, the ceramist has a choice of two methods to incorporate the incisal edge maverick into the restoration: the use of body modifiers or stains.

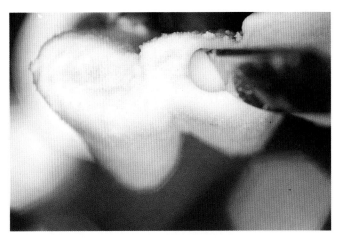

Fig 4-23 Applying body modifier to scooped out incisal edge. In cases where the dentin has discolored only at the incisal edge due to the complete wearing away of the enamel in this area, the surface maverick duplicating method is recommended; the entire dentin is built to full contour (hue-chroma dimension) and covered over completely with enamel porcelain. When scooping out the incisal area, care must be taken to leave a wall of enamel porcelain so that a definite boundary is established between it and the embedded modifier. The depth of the scooped out area will depend on needed color concentration and available space.

Body Modifiers (Fig 4-23)

A portion of the incisodentin is scooped out, with care being taken to leave the enamel porcelain intact; this could measure from 0.2 to 1 mm in depth, depending on the maverick color and needed concentration. (The higher the concentration, the more depth required, whereas less color concentration requires less depth.) The scooped out area is filled with the selected maverick color (body modifier). Care must be taken that the original porcelain buildup remains in a semiwet state when the modifier is added. Adding porcelain to a dry buildup could create porosity, weakness, crazing, or flaking in the porcelain during firing. The newly added modifier (which has been mixed with the proper amount of neutral porcelain to

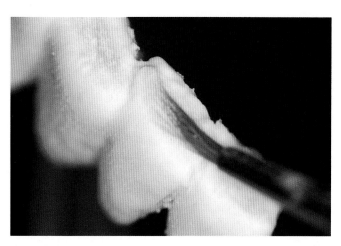

Fig 4-24 Stains can be used to satisfy needed color at the incisal edge of anterior restorations. It is applied directly to the body and enamel buildup so that a definite demarcation is developed between the dentin and enamel. Stain can also be used with embedded modifiers when more color concentration or accents are needed to comply with CTC.

obtain needed concentration) should be carefully vibrated into position, taking care not to disturb the outer enamel porcelain shell that forms a definite demarcation between dentin and enamel. After firing, only a minimal amount of contouring is required since the needed length was established during porcelain buildup and maintained with the enamel porcelain. Compensation for shrinkage must be provided during porcelain buildup; however, the amount of overbuilding will vary with the brand of porcelain used and the amount of condensing. During functional contouring, there is no danger of color loss on the incisal edge because of its depth. Wear facets and any other needed contouring for esthetic harmony should be included before final glazing takes place.

Stains

Another method for incorporating incisal edge maverick is by using stain instead of body modi-

fiers. The entire porcelain buildup is the same as with the body modifier technique. Instead of scooping out the incisal dentin, it is left intact and the proper stain (corresponding to the selected maverick color) is applied to it. It is important to remember that although modifiers are desaturated by mixing them with neutral porcelain, stains are desaturated with liquid medium. Both techniques simply move the color particles far enough apart to produce the needed saturated version for the selected maverick color. When applying the stain, care must be taken to maintain the demarcation between dentin and enamel (Fig 4-24).

The stain method is used in cases where the incisal length leaves little or no room for embedding modifier. The advantage of using stain is that its high potency allows the ceramist to obtain high color concentrations in very thin areas. By the same token, their high potency could produce overconcentration of color. Care should be taken to desaturate the stain to the precise concentration necessary to duplicate the selected maverick color. It should also be applied to the semiwet porcelain with sufficient vibration so that the stain liquid medium and the porcelain buildup liquid become thoroughly mixed. To violate this procedure could result in porosity and fracture at the stain-porcelain junction.

Yet even guaranteeing sufficient vibration, color depth is usually shallow. This limits the amount of allowable incisal adjustment after firing; care must be taken during porcelain buildup to compensate for shrinkage, eliminating the need for excessive incisal adjustment.

The amount of available incisal length will dictate which color source to use: body modifier or stain. The general rule is to use modifiers in cases with adequate length and to use stains in cases of insufficient length.

The incisal edge maverick technique so far has been applied to cases that encompass the four tooth color dimensions (hue, chroma, maverick, and value). There are cases, however, that fall into the category of maverick and enamel, which means that the entire dentin is made up of a maverick color, covered completely with enamel. In cases such as this, the enamel on the incisal edge has been worn to the point that the underlying dentin is completely exposed, revealing just two tooth color dimensions: maverick and value. This simplifies the entire procedure in that the entire body buildup is made up of the maverick color found on the incisal edge of the tooth. There is no need to add incisal color; the color is found throughout the entire tooth, as it will be in the fabricated restoration (see Figs 4-10a to i).

Whichever the case might be, when incisal edge maverick is detected, its concentration must be measured and incorporated into the restoration in order to maintain esthetic harmony.

Enamel Hypocalcification

Enamel hypocalcification occurs when there is subnormal calcification of the enamel and it materializes in the form of opaque white spots usually found in the incisal third of tooth enamel. These areas of hypocalcification range from subtle, almost unnoticeable specks, to large, very obvious white opaque splotches. Although they are generally found in the incisal third, it is not uncommon to find them in other areas of the enamel.

Enamel development occurs in two separate phases: matrix formation and maturation. Irregularities that occur in enamel depend entirely on the phase of development the enamel was in when a disturbance occurred. If the matrix formation is affected, enamel *hypoplasia* will result. If there is a deficiency in the mineral content of the enamel during maturation, *hypocalcification* of the enamel will develop.

Cause of Hypocalcification

Causes of hypocalcification can be classified as: (1) systemic, (2) local, and (3) hereditary. Mottled enamel is an example of systemic enamel hypocalcification. A high fluoride content in the water will cause a deficiency in calcification. Fluoride hypocalcification is found in certain areas (endemic) where the drinking water contains more than one part of fluoride per 1 million parts of water. The same local causes that might affect the formation of enamel can disrupt maturation. If the injury occurs in the formation stage of enamel development, hypoplasia of the enamel will result; an injury during the maturation stage will cause a deficiency in calcification.

The hereditary type of hypocalcification is characterized by the formation of a normal amount of enamel matrix that does not fully mature. Such teeth, if investigated before or shortly after eruption, are normal in shape. Their surfaces do not have the luster of normal enamel, however, and they appear dull and the enamel is opaque. In very extreme cases, the hypocalcified areas of the enamel are soft and could discolor. These areas are easily abraded by mastication and can pull off in layers. When this occurs, the teeth will be rough and discolored due to the exposed underlying dentin, which is spongelike and vulnerable to stain and wear.

Detecting and Measuring Hypocalcification

In most cases, in spite of hypocalcification, teeth are otherwise healthy and only a few require restorative treatment. As previously stated, the extent of this irregularity ranges from just a few insignificant white specs to large areas of opacity. In any event, when these areas of opacity are detected, they must be incorporated in the restoration if esthetic harmony is to be maintained. During detection, two important factors must be considered. First, these spots or areas of hypocalcification will vary in intensity from time to time due to physiological conditions and breathing habits of the patient. So called mouth breathers tend to exhibit this condition more than others. In some patients, the intensity will be great and will linger for weeks, then for no apparent reason will subside and in a few cases disappear for a short period of time. Second, during tooth preparation, the teeth will tend to dry out because of absent normal saliva activity. The intensity of the opaque areas will increase, displaying this irregularity more than is usual during normal oral function. For these reasons, it is imperative that during duplication these hypocalcified areas be subtly included so that when they become less noticeable in the natural dentition, the restoration will not stand out. It is a good practice, therefore, to purposely underemphasize hypocalcification in the restoration.

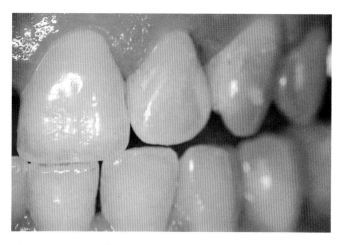

Fig 4-25 Maxillary central and lateral incisors displaying several degrees of hypocalcification. Hypocalcification located in the incisal third of the central incisor is so subtle, it might go unnoticed under normal scrutiny. White stain is stippled lightly into the dentin layer or mixed with dentin porcelain and placed in prescribed areas of the restoration. This is completely covered with a thin layer of dentin, then finally with a layer of enamel porcelain. The lateral incisor exhibits a more pronounced degree of hypocalcification in the mesial and incisal third. To achieve this in a restoration, white stain is brushed lightly over the semiwet dentin buildup. The only covering should be a layer of enamel porcelain, which will result in a slightly more intense result than that found in the central incisor.

Duplicating Hypocalcification

The ideal material for duplicating hypocalcification in a restoration is white stain. Because of its white opacity and strong potency, it can be manipulated into any one of several stages of porcelain buildup. To be natural looking, the stain should be embedded into the pre-fired porcelain, not added as a surface stain after firing. It is much easier to control location and concentration of the stain deposits during porcelain buildup. The needed effect, location, and concentration will determine the method for incorporating the stain into the restoration.

Most subtle (Fig 4-25). The most subtle of all the methods is to mix a portion of white stain with the prescribed dentin porcelain (hue-chroma dimension) for a particular case; this permits you to dilute its effect to the very minimum. The mixture is set aside until the dentin buildup is completed. At that time, areas of dentin porcelain are scooped out and replaced with the premixed stain. The original buildup should be in a semiwet state when adding the premixed stain. The subtlety is further extended by the enamel porcelain overlay.

When properly executed, even though the white stain is thoroughly buried, this technique will produce very subtle white opaque spots in prescribed areas of the restoration. Furthermore, due to the higher potency of white stain, these areas will appear to be on the surface rather than beneath it.

Subtle (Fig 4-25). In cases that require more emphasis, the white stain is applied directly to the surface of the dentin buildup. This method requires the dentin buildup to be properly contoured, with adequate room for enamel porcelain, so that only absolute minimal grinding is necessary after firing. Even though the stain is applied lightly, if care is not taken to control its dilution, the results may be too pronounced. Dilute the stain with liquid medium to cut down its intensity before applying it to the surface of the semiwet dentin porcelain. Use vibration to incorporate the stain and liquid medium

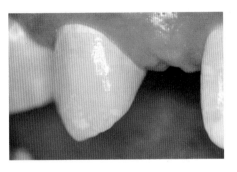

Fig 4-26

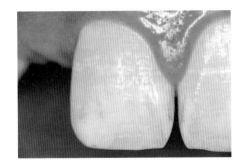

Fig 4-27

Fig 4-26   A more noticeable hypocalcification area is displayed in the incisal third of the maxillary right canine (also gingival third). When incorporating stain into the body buildup, care must be taken to keep the additions to a minimum so as to prevent the possibility of disrupting the coefficient of expansion between the porcelain and the metal substructure.

Fig 4-27   Maxillary right central incisor with bold hypocalcification area (mottled enamel). In cases such as this, the area of hypocalcification is usually quite large, sometimes covering as much as 75% of the tooth's surface. The white stain should be mixed with stain liquid medium in order to keep the color particles together. When applying the stain to the enamel porcelain, slight vibration is necessary to incorporate the stain liquid medium with the porcelain buildup liquid to prevent porosity or possible porcelain fracture.

with the porcelain. While the dentin-stain buildup is still in a semiwet state, apply the enamel porcelain to fulfill the required contour of the restoration, taking care not to disturb the stain distribution. After final contour and glaze, the restoration should reveal a subtle display of hypocalcification that is pronounced enough to be recognized but subtle enough not to be conspicuous.

Noticeable (Fig 4-26).   For a slightly more noticeable hypocalcification effect, the white stain can be brought closer to the surface. A mixture of white stain and enamel porcelain is prepared and set aside. The enamel buildup is completed to full contour, and using a fine brush, the prepared mixture is applied to locations throughout the enamel layer. This desaturated mixture is controllable because its strength is indirectly proportional

to the amount of enamel porcelain the white stain is added to. That is, the more noticeable the results, the less enamel porcelain needs to be mixed with a given amount of white stain. For less noticeable results, more enamel porcelain should be added to a given amount of white stain. When in doubt as to the strength of the mixture, fire a sample tab. Formula changes can be made accordingly. Do not overbuild the restoration, for this could require excessive grinding, especially in cases where precise labial thickness and incisal contour and position are a major concern for a successful result. Any amount of grinding over absolute minimal requirements could remove the embedded areas of hypocalcification.

Bold (Fig 4-27).   Cases of extreme hypocalcification found in the natural dentition should be toned

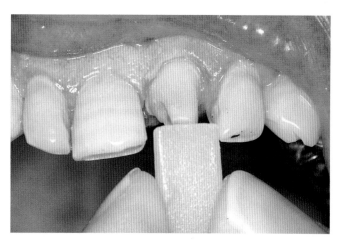

Fig 4-28a

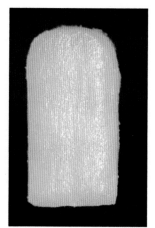

Fig 4-28b

Fig 4-28a   An example of disorganized color, and use of a customized color tab to measure the maverick dimension. Note the bands of color and how they do not conform with normal tooth color location. The bands of color in this case are actually caused by areas of very thin enamel where underlying color projects through.

Fig 4-28b   A sample CTC tab that shows exact color, concentration, and location can be used throughout the entire laboratory procedure when restoring a dentition that shows disorganized color. The tab can be taken to the mouth and compared to the tooth before preparation or compared to unprepared teeth in the vicinity of the tooth to be restored. In the laboratory, porcelain application can be made using the tab as a guide.

down and de-emphasized in the restoration whenever possible. This can be easily accomplished where several units are involved and especially where a full quadrant is being restored. There are cases, however, where it is imperative to incorporate these hypocalcification areas in a bold manner so as to match adjacent teeth. This is best accomplished by brush-dabbing areas of decalcification with a premixed preparation of white stain and liquid medium directly onto the surface of enamel porcelain buildup. This should be vibrated slightly to embed the stain into the enamel layer. The fired restoration will show areas of pronounced whitish opaqueness that will hopefully blend with those areas found in the natural dentition. In this method, it is important that

a minimum of grinding take place during the final contour stage before glazing. As unsightly as this irregularity may seem, to eliminate it from a restoration that must have it to match adjacent teeth could produce an unacceptable result.

Irregularities Over the Entire Labial Surface

Although most irregularities can usually be found in certain areas of the tooth (ie, gingival, middle, and incisal third), some monopolize the entire labial surface. Most of the labial and buccal irregularities can be traced back to early tooth devel-

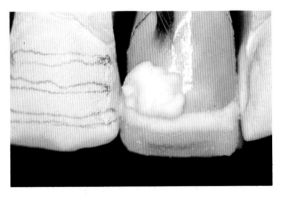

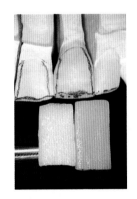

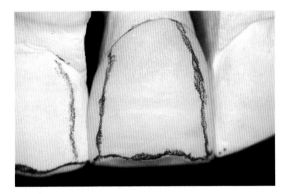

Fig 4-28c   **Fig 4-28d**   **Fig 4-28e**

Fig 4-28c   Bands of porcelain are applied over prefired maverick color (maverick over opaque method) to comply with the color formation found in the maxillary right central incisor. Although a color pattern has been drawn on the master working model, it is not necessary or recommended to follow the exact color location found on the right central incisor; color location should vary somewhat between the two central incisors. Note the porcelain being applied over a previously fired shell that has established the incisal edge. A thin layer of enamel covers the entire restoration before firing.

Fig 4-28d   Restoration contoured and ready for glaze being compared to the two customized color tabs (maverick and enamel). Note the incisal edge position and contour developed by the opposing dentition.

Fig 4-28e   Restoration ready for aluminum oxide spray, steam cleaning, and glaze. At this stage it can be compared with the sample CTC tab to verify color and location.

opment; the histological aspect has much to do with how the tooth reflects its health or lack of it by displaying certain irregularities over its entire surface.

Disorganized Color (Figs 4-28a to e)

When we refer to normal tooth color, we usually visualize the tooth as having color distributed logically throughout; that is, more concentrated at the gingival third, less concentrated at the middle third because of greater enamel thickness, and very little color, if any, at the incisal third and buccal cusp tips. Most ceramic restorations are designed according to this concept, as are most artificial teeth used for dentures. However, there are teeth that do not follow this rule. Instead of exhibiting color and color concentrations in the three logical locations, the labial or buccal surface shows disorganized color. For example, the gingival color may be less concentrated than the middle third, or the incisal third may show more color than either the middle or gingival third. Teeth having disorganized color are usually healthy; the unusual color distribution is attributed to enamel thickness and its relationship to the underlying dentin. Thin areas of enamel permit more dentin color to project through; thicker areas of enamel block out the dentin influence. These areas tend to be mesiodistal rather than incisogingival. Patient age does not seem to be a factor, which lends to

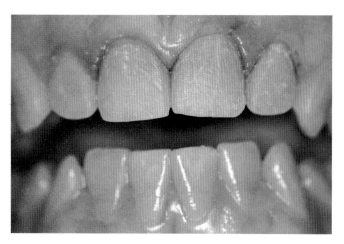

Fig 4-29 Young patient with permanent tooth discoloration due to the ingestion of tetracycline during tooth development. Discoloration usually involves the entire dentin.

the theory that disorganized color evolves during tooth development. The mesiodistal configuration confirms this theory.

A simple diagram should be drawn for the ceramist to point out color concentration and location, and a customized tooth color guide should give exact measurements. Or, a photograph or slide can be taken to show the color *location* (it is impossible to rely on photography for color duplication).

The presence of disorganized color actually simplifies detection, measurement, and duplication of CTC. Hue, chroma, and maverick are more obvious due to the thin areas of enamel, hence the guess work is eliminated and in most cases the enamel need not be removed before measuring the tooth color dimensions. Furthermore, even though color configuration can vary somewhat between the tooth and restoration, the closer the resemblance, the more acceptable it will be. For this reason, a sample CTC tab should be constructed before the tooth is prepared. The tab is built to full contour before firing. It can be completed in a very short time, with relatively little

effort, and sent back to the dentist for evaluation before the tooth is prepared. Whether this procedure is accomplished in one appointment or two, the extra effort is well worth it; the dentist can point out needed changes that must be made for the final restoration. This not only improves dentist-laboratory communication and relationship, it creates more confidence between dentist and patient by helping to eliminate possible remakes due to incorrect CTC duplication.

Tetracycline Influence

Another irregularity not necessarily associated with unhealthy dentition is one that manifests itself in the form of erratic tooth discoloration and is brought about by tetracycline ingestion during childhood. When tetracycline is taken during tooth development, the fluorescent tetracycline particles may become incorporated into the dentin during dentin calcification, resulting in varying degrees of fluorescence. This usually results in permanent tooth discoloration, ranging from low values of yellow to orange to brown.

Tetracycline influence on tooth color varies from being mild to unsightly. Although there is no evidence that it hinders tooth development or causes physical or chemical damage, the discoloration can be damaging psychologically; a person can suffer much embarrassment during adolescence and even during adulthood (Fig 4-29).

In recent years, there have been many advancements in bonding techniques and improved materials that have proven useful for treating cases of tetracycline discoloration and other tooth deformities. There are some limitations to bonding, however, and often the dentist must resort to a less conservative approach for solving the problem: the metal ceramic restoration. This involves full tooth preparation with a lifetime commitment to tooth coverage.

Cases of tetracycline discoloration fall into two categories as far as CTC is concerned. First is the "must duplicate" category, which usually involves

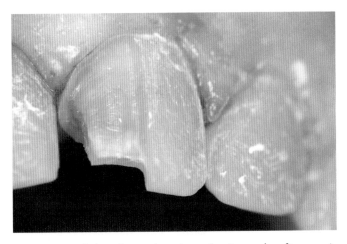

Fig 4-30 Color dimension detection is made after semi-preparing maxillary left central incisor. Removing enamel from half of the tooth to the dentinoenamel junction reveals the color found in the dentin as a result of tetracycline. Comparing the prepared half to the unprepared half reveals the influence the enamel has on CTC. In most cases where less than a quadrant of teeth are to be restored, it is almost imperative to duplicate CTC exactly in order to maintain color harmony with the surrounding teeth. When a segment is restored entirely for cosmetic reasons, color alterations can be made.

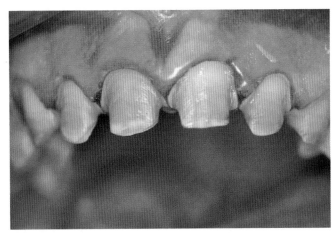

Fig 4-31 The six maxillary anterior teeth prepared and made ready to be restored. The purpose for restoration is for cosmetic improvement, therefore the entire segment is included; it is not necessary to duplicate the colors exactly as detected. The colors in the restoration should be more pleasing than those located in the dentin.

just one tooth or a few teeth. In this case the CTC must be duplicated exactly so that the restoration harmonizes with the natural dentition. Second is the "cosmetically motivated" category, in which the sole reason for treatment is to improve esthetics. Each category has an entirely different approach to obtaining ideal CTC.

"Must Duplicate" Category

In spite of the fact that the maverick dimension plays a prime role and is the most outstanding color dimension in cases such as this, it is interesting to note that in many cases, the basic dentin color (hue-chroma) is quite pleasant, and to overlook this could leave a void in the duplicating process. The extent of unaffected dentin depends on (1) the age at which the child was treated

with tetracycline, (2) the length of treatment, and (3) the development stage the teeth were in during treatment.

Detection. Family color and location must be determined. The hue and chroma sections of the CTC guide are used to determine the basic hue and further refinement of the remaining unaffected dentin. Too often, this dimension is overlooked and the ceramist is tempted to merely duplicate the maverick dimension. Remember that the CTC is the combination of *all* the color found beneath the enamel layer. To eliminate a dimension, regardless what degree it plays, is to derail a precise duplication. After the hue-chroma family and location have been found, the maverick dimension is located and basic family color determined (Figs 4-30 and 4-31).

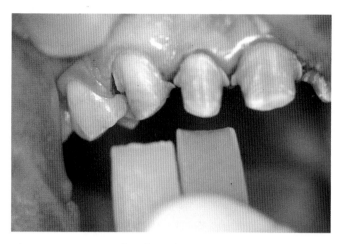

Fig 4-32 Maverick color tabs are used to determine the family color in the teeth to be restored. If an exact color duplication is required, as would be the case when restoring just one tooth, the selected tabs would dictate the colors needed for the CTC. In this case, however, where the entire segment will be restored, the detected colors can be diluted with neutral porcelain, thus giving the restoration a more pleasant CTC (the hue-chroma dimension was not included in this case because of the overpowering maverick influence).

Measurement. When areas of dentin with normal color are detected (color that falls into the hue-chroma dimension), the hue guide from the CTC guide is used to determine the hue dimension. The color family selected during detection will determine from which color group the tab will be pulled (yellow, orange, gray, etc). For example, if the basic family color is yellow, in the Vita System a tab from the "B" series most closely matching the dentin (hue) is pulled. If the hue tab matches the dentin perfectly, there is no need for further refinement. However, if the selected tab matches the basic hue but is too concentrated, the chroma guide must be brought into play.

Next, the maverick guide is used to measure the maverick deposits found throughout the tooth. In cases involving tetracycline influence, it is not uncommon to find several different color families with varying degrees of saturation. It is usually necessary to use the maverick guide, selecting the

tab in its most saturated form. Many cases will require highly concentrated tabs, whereas others will call for some degree of dilution.

Finally, the last dimension, value, is measured. The value tab that matches the enamel of the tooth will be the tab that dictates the amount of gray needed to be added to enamel porcelain in order to duplicate the exact brightness of the tooth in the restoration. The mistake often made when lowering the value in cases that need more gray than normal, is to add gray modifier to the dentin porcelain buildup. Regardless how low the value may be, the hue-chroma dimension must be maintained and unaltered. To add gray modifier to the dentin porcelain buildup will indeed alter the hue-chroma dimension and cancel out the needed effect this dimension contributes to the CTC. Responsibility for regulating value should be delegated to the enamel porcelain, which covers the restoration completely, thus distributing its effect throughout.

At this point, the three tabs, along with a diagram and any other needed information, can now be sent to the laboratory for duplication (Fig 4-32).

Duplication. The prescribed method for duplicating the four tooth color dimensions in a tetracycline case is embedded maverick because maverick color family and concentration can be more easily controlled and more accurately placed using this than using any of the other methods for duplication.

1. *Opaque.* The opaque is applied in two separate firings, the first being a thin opaque wash made up of the opaque assigned to the hue-chroma and the second consisting of portions of opaque, dentin, and body modifier (see chapter 3).

2. *Dentin buildup.* As mentioned, the embedded maverick method for duplication works well. This method permits the placement of the maverick colors into the dentin buildup in exact locations determined during color detection. This duplicating method is preferred over the maverick buildup method because it places the colors closer to the

surface, thus increasing its ability to display its effect, as opposed to burying the colors deep into the restoration and covering it over with dentin porcelain, as found in the maverick buildup method. In most cases such as this, the maverick colors will be covered with enamel porcelain only.

When attempting to match the maverick colors exactly with no color improvement, it is advisable to fire the hue-chroma-maverick (dentin) and value (enamel) separately. This enables the ceramist to compare the selected CTC tabs to the fired dentin before the enamel covering is made and permits any necessary changes to be made before final firing. The firing temperature is slightly lower than the transition layer firing and should be maintained according to the manufacturer's specifications.

3. *Enamel.* The enamel layer will also be somewhat unorthodox in that it may be necessary to add certain irregularities not normally found there. Areas of hypoplasia and hypocalcification are not uncommon in cases of tetracycline discoloration and should be included where needed. Incorporating white and gray stain in needed degrees of concentration will usually satisfy this requirement. The stains are applied to the prefired porcelain buildup after being desaturated to desired strength with liquid medium. Care must be taken to: (1) not add stain to dry enamel porcelain; the enamel buildup must be in a semiwet state so that it will not draw liquid from the stain mixture — this could cause porosity and fracture, and (2) slightly vibrate stain into enamel porcelain to ensure complete mixture of stain medium and buildup liquid or distilled water. Vibrating should be kept to a minimum, taking care to not spread the stain into inappropriate areas.

After adequate drying time, the case is fired to an eggshell finish, contoured, and glazed. If care is taken to not overbuild, only a minimal amount of contouring is required, thus lessening the possibility of grinding away ingredients necessary for CTC. Careful consideration should be taken to incorporate the same degree of texture and glaze as found in the natural dentition.

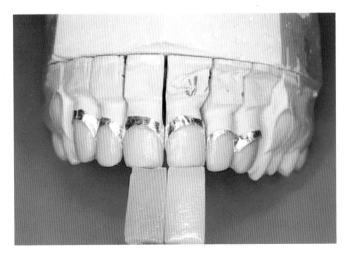

Fig 4-33 Dentin buildup using a desaturated version of the original two selected maverick color tabs. When improving CTC for esthetic reasons, it is important to maintain the original family color and not to dilute the colors so much that they cease to harmonize with the surrounding dentition. After confirming the fired dentin layer with the desaturated maverick color tabs, the enamel layer is applied and fired, after which the restorations are contoured and glazed.

While this technique is prescribed for duplicating tetracycline influence precisely as detected and measured, a technique for softening or toning down its effects should be considered and used where such color improvements are called for.

If the treatment plan is formulated primarily for cosmetic reasons, the most important concern is that the final restoration harmonize with the remaining natural dentition. To harmonize does not necessarily mean to duplicate exactly as previously described. Harmonizing permits change with some leeway for color and contour, the only requirement being sufficient blending with the remaining dentition so as to give no sign of artificiality (Fig 4-33). In order to comply with this requirement, it is important to keep the same color family in the hue-chroma and maverick dimension. For example, should the hue-chroma dimension be classified as being in the orange-brown

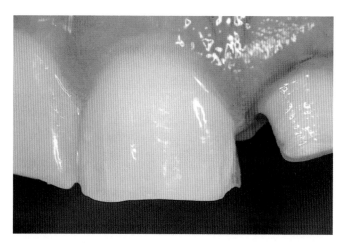

Fig 4-34 Maxillary right central incisor of a middle-aged patient with several vertical craze lines, the most obvious being located at the distal third. Its worn incisal edge is a good indication that the cause for this minor irregularity is the abnormal wear patterns brought about by the mandibular anterior teeth. As the patient ages, the number of enamel craze lines will probably increase and discolor, becoming more recognizable. The restored left central incisor should include several subtle craze lines, placed approximately in the same location as the right central incisor.

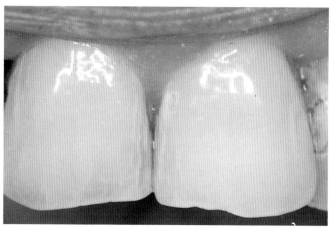

Fig 4-35 Maxillary central incisors displaying more advanced stages of enamel craze lines as compared to those found in Fig 4-34. With age and wear, the amount of craze lines will increase, as will their discoloration. Restorations in the vicinity of these teeth should include several craze lines with a hint of color but not necessarily as pronounced as those found in the central incisors; patients usually prefer that the restored teeth blend with remaining dentition yet show some esthetic improvement.

color family, it must not be augmented to the yellow or gray family. Likewise, if the maverick dimension is considered yellow, it should not be altered to an orange or brown family. The color families must not be changed, merely softened. This is accomplished with the addition of neutral porcelain.

The amount of color softening should be decided during color dimension detection and measurement, at which time the patient is informed as to the intended treatment plan. Comparisons should be made with the selected CTC tabs that measure the color dimensions precisely with those to be used for the fabricated restoration. When the primary reason for treatment is for cosmetic improvement, the patient should be included during case planning to ensure complete understanding of the intended results. The patient should be encouraged to volunteer as much input as possi-

ble so the dentist knows exactly what the patient expects. If these expectations exceed the proposed final results, due to limitations, the dentist should point out these facts, explaining these limitations and stating basic guidelines that dictate what can be done. Patients whose primary interest is cosmetic improvement are usually very critical; to prevent disappointment, a complete understanding of the intended results must be made before initiating the case.

Crazed Enamel

Enamel craze lines can be found in many teeth. Although they are more common in the middle aged and elderly, this condition can also exist in younger people (Figs 4-34 and 4-35). Crazing is aggravated by excessive stresses placed upon

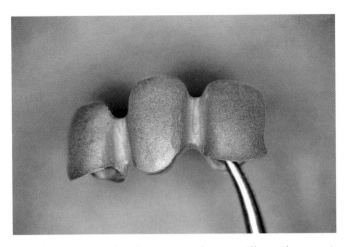

Fig 4-36a Metal substructure for maxillary three-unit restoration ready for opaque and body porcelain application. The maverick-over-opaque method will be used (see chapter 3).

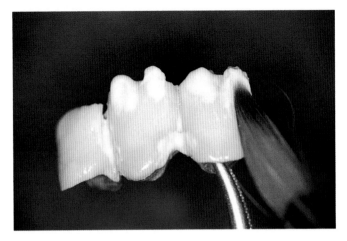

Fig 4-36b Applying body color modifiers over the maverick dimension that was previously fired over the transition layer. The color family and concentration of these colors are dictated by the surrounding dentition. Craze lines are not developed during this application.

these teeth, and severity of the condition ranges from single, almost unnoticeable to multiple, very pronounced lines. Depending on eating and drinking habits, as well as the extent of oral hygiene, these craze lines may exhibit some degree of color. Coffee, tea, tobacco, and certain foods lend to intense coloration. Craze lines usually extend vertically over the full length of the tooth. Conditions such as bruxism, malocclusion, or any other condition that causes excessive or abnormal stresses to be placed on certain teeth provide the ideal environment for this to occur.

Like most other so-called irregularities, the question arises as to whether crazing should be included in the restoration. This depends on how many units are in the restoration and where they are located. Anteriorly, it is imperative that some amount of this irregularity be included; if not, like most other common irregularities, the restoration will not harmonize with the natural dentition. When six anterior teeth are involved, the craze lines could be completely excluded, or included with less emphasis. The patient should be asked to decide.

Duplication (Figs 4-36 to 4-38)

The duplication method prescribed for each case varies with the needs of that case. The basic procedure for duplicating craze lines requires vertical layering of porcelain, as opposed to standard porcelain buildup. Although craze lines are located in the enamel layer of natural dentition, they are duplicated in the dentin porcelain layer during vertical layering then are covered over completely with enamel porcelain. Even in the most severe cases, which require high concentration of lines and color, all of the required duplication can take place during the dentin porcelain buildup. The enamel porcelain covering promotes depth and subtlety in the restoration.

The crazed effect can be obtained by separating vertical layers of dentin porcelain with ultrathin layers of stain. The stains most commonly used in this technique fall in certain color families. Along with white and gray, which are colorless, yellow, orange, and brown in various concentrations and combinations are used.

In early stages, crazing is usually colorless and

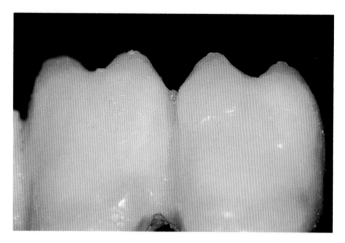

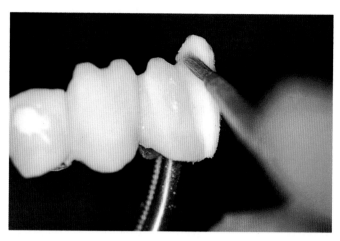

Fig 4-36c Fired incisal body modifiers. This layering supplies needed maverick color deposits to the restoration and also helps to recontour the incisal third and hide the crescent shape of the metal substructure. Areas between color deposits are left for transparent porcelain, which will be deposited during the next application of porcelain. The recontoured incisal third is not only especially helpful in preventing the substructure from showing through, it also leaves areas free for needed incisal transparency.

Fig 4-36d Incorporating a subtle orange-brown craze line during dentin buildup (vertical layering). A very thin, diluted mixture of orange and brown stain is applied to a vertical wall of dentin porcelain (transparent incisally) and will go almost unnoticed in the restoration. It will typify a craze line that has just begun to discolor.

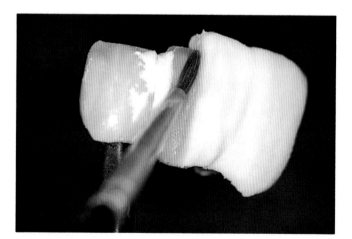

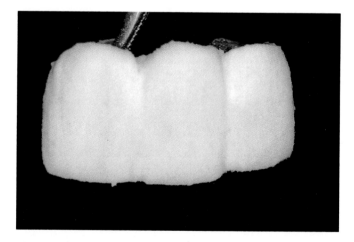

Fig 4-36e A more concentrated mixture of orange and brown stain is applied to give the effect of an aged craze line that can be discolored or a subtle check line that shows through a separation in the enamel. As craze lines age, they tend to discolor. Therefore, in restorations that need them, several degrees of discoloration may be necessary (ie, whitish-gray to orange-brown). The number of lines and the color of each are determined by the surrounding dentition.

Fig 4-36f Complete dentin buildup using vertical layering. The enamel porcelain could be applied at this stage and fired together with the dentin; however, in restorations where complicated irregularities are involved, the dentin should be fired before the enamel application so that any needed adjustments can be made before the enamel is applied. When this occurs, sufficient room over the entire surface of the restoration must be left to accommodate the enamel layer. A thin separation is made between units to allow for equal shrinkage of each.

Fig 4-36g   Fired, vertically layered dentin of the restoration, revealing craze lines and other needed irregularities incorporated into the body porcelain buildup. Note the equal amount of shrinkage that occurred between units due to the separations made before firing. This is important in that it (1) permits each unit to absorb an equal amount of shrinkage, thus eliminating the possibility of stresses in the porcelain; (2) develops a stronger porcelain because of the compacting of porcelain particles; (3) enhances the color by pulling color oxides closer together; and (4) makes room interproximally if more color is needed in the form of deposits or discolored restorations.

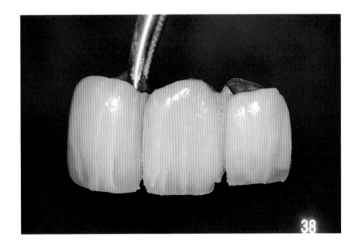

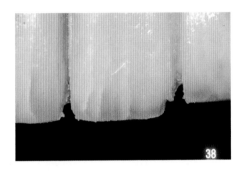

Fig 4-36h

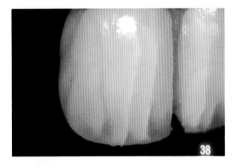

Fig 4-36i

Fig 4-36h   Magnification of fired restoration showing vertical craze lines with varying degrees of intensity. Note subtle orange-brown check line near center of the left central incisor (refer to Fig 4-36e). Also, note incisal transparency and maverick frame that was developed during craze line formation.

Fig 4-36i   Maxillary right central incisor restoration. Note two white craze lines with high concentrations of white stain. Diluted gray stain applied as an extension to the white stain internally creates a shadow effect and adds authenticity to this irregularity. Note interproximal color and space made available during shrinkage for more needed color. If there are no corrections to be made, the next porcelain application will be enamel, which should cover the entire restoration. Even though crazing occurs in the enamel of the tooth, it should be placed in the dentin of the restoration to ensure subtlety.

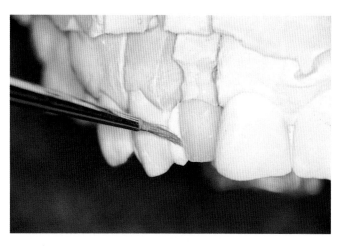

Fig 4-37a Diluted white stain is applied to a vertical wall of dentin porcelain on a maxillary right lateral incisor. A very diluted gray stain is added as an extension to create a shadow (refer to Fig 4-36i). The stains are mixed with liquid stain medium (rather than distilled water) for better handling. When applying to semiwet dentin porcelain, slight vibration is necessary to incorporate the stain liquid medium with the procelain buildup liquid; this will prevent porosity and/or fracture.

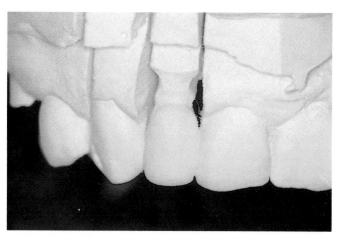

Fig 4-37b A thin layer of enamel porcelain is applied over craze lines, and dentin and is contoured to exact specifications except for a slight increase in length and mesial and distal contacts to compensate for shrinkage. Overbuilding porcelain creates the need for excessive grinding and shaping after firing, which could remove needed irregularities and color.

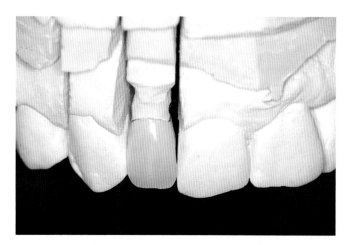

Fig 4-37c Completed restoration on master working model. Satin texture and glaze obtained by hand polishing after minimum furnace glaze. Craze lines are visible but not overbearing.

subtle. This can be duplicated easily with white stain with a very dilute gray to assimilate a shadow. This is accomplished using the deep stain maverick method. The early stages of crazing are the most subtle, and care should be taken during duplication to bury the lines deep into the dentin.

The white and gray stains are mixed with stain liquid medium and set aside. The dentin porcelain is mixed, as are the selected maverick color or colors necessary to complete the CTC. Even though irregularities are important to consider and should be included in the restoration, the four tooth color dimensions are of prime concern. Therefore, the crazing, like other irregularities, will be incorporated into the restoration according to the method used to duplicate the CTC.

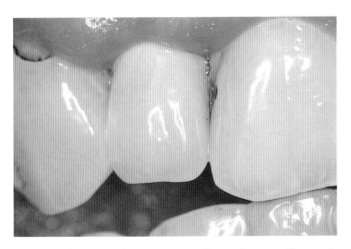

Fig 4-37d Seated restoration. Three-day recall reveals improved gingival health in spite of a metal margin. A fine bevel and well-glazed porcelain in this area ensure an adequate seal and healthy tissue.

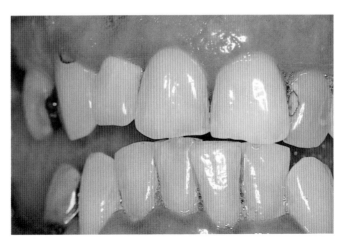

Fig 4-37e The seated maxillary right lateral incisor restoration harmonizes well with the surrounding dentition. In cases such as this where tooth color is not uniform throughout, it is advisable to select color and irregularities from several teeth (ie, subtle craze lines were taken from the right central incisor and colors were taken from both maxillary and mandibular anterior teeth). The restoration should blend with all 12 anterior teeth.

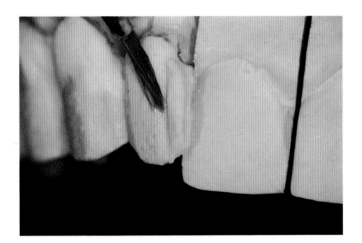

Fig 4-38a Maxillary master working model with four-unit restoration in the process of fabrication. Craze lines are applied during vertical layering of dentin porcelain. Thin stain (white and gray) application with a quick, light stroke ensures a natural-appearing restoration. Excess stain should be carefully brushed away to prevent unwanted color deposits. Note modification at gingival third that will eventually be covered with dentin porcelain.

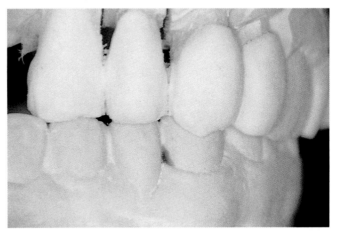

Fig 4-38b Completed dentin buildup (vertical layering) with incorporated craze lines. Room is left for enamel porcelain that could be applied at this stage or after the dentin is fired. Lateral excursions and protrusive movement are registered before firing, to ensure proper function. interproximal slices are made to allow each unit to shrink uniformly.

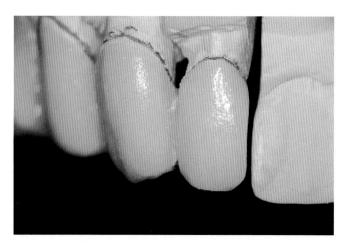

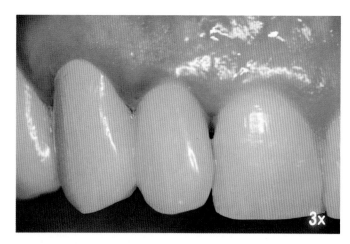

Fig 4-38c Fired dentin. Note subtle craze lines in canine and lateral incisor and interproximal shrinkage. The basic family color was out of range of the hue-chroma shade guide, making it necessary to use the maverick-and-enamel duplicating method. A thin layer of enamel porcelain will completely cover the restoration.

Fig 4-38d Fired enamel layer is contoured and glazed. Note how the subtle craze lines project through the enamel layer in a natural fashion and how well they blend with those in the right central incisor, even though they are located in the dentin of the restoration but in the enamel of the natural dentition.

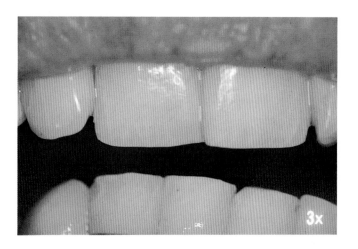

Fig 4-38e Maxillary right lateral incisor restoration as compared to maxillary and mandibular anterior teeth. It is important that a restoration blend not only with immediate adjacent teeth, but also with all others in the general vicinity. This often requires incorporating features from several teeth into a restoration, as was also found in Fig 4-37c.

Colored Check Line (Fig 4-39)

A colored check line, similar to an enamel craze line, is a vertical line extending from the gingival third to the incisal third of the tooth. The two cases differ, however, in that a check line is usually more pronounced and exhibits individuality rather than being one of a cluster of craze lines. It is often found as a distinct separation in the enamel, unlike the smooth, flawless enamel surface found in enamel craze lines.

In duplicating a colored check line, stain is placed vertically during the dentin buildup with varying thickness and intensity and is usually formed in conjunction with an obvious separation in the enamel. However, it is not necessary to use the vertical layering technique to achieve this irregularity; it can be placed into the restoration after the dentin and enamel have been built to full contour.

Duplicating a check line is uncomplicated when used with any of the eight methods for duplicating CTC because the line is placed by embedding the proper color after dissecting the unfired porcelain buildup. As in any other restoration where stain is used with unfired porcelain, the stain is mixed with liquid medium and applied to a semiwet dentin porcelain. Slight vibration is required to ensure complete mixing of the stain liquid medium with the porcelain buildup liquid.

In restorations requiring the maverick and enamel method for duplicating CTC, the underlying dentin (made up of body modifier) can be fabricated such that it projects the check line color through the enamel separation. This is accomplished by forming a vertical separation in the enamel porcelain while applying it to the underlying maverick body buildup. The separation width is varied to accommodate needed intensity.

Mottled Enamel

High fluorine concentrations found in food and water ingested during enamel calcification can

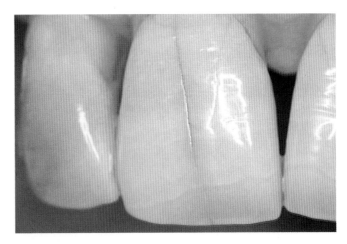

Fig 4-39 Maxillary right central incisor displaying a check line. A check line is usually brought about by a separation in the enamel that permits discoloration to take place. It could also develop from an aged craze line that has created an access through the enamel. The color ranges from orange to brown (usually a combination of the two) and can be incorporated into the restoration either during vertical layering (see Fig 4-38b) when a subtle result is needed, or it can be applied closer to the surface upon completing the porcelain buildup. Where the entire dentin is in the maverick color range, a slight separation in the enamel porcelain before glazing will produce the same result.

cause mottled enamel. This has been found to prevail especially in areas where the drinking water has an overabundance of fluorine. Extra-high concentrations of fluorine are believed to cause metabolic alterations in the ameloblasts during enamel formation, which results in a defective matrix and improper calcification. Fluorosis is classified as mild, moderate, or severe, depending on the amount of fluorides ingested during amelogenesis.

Mild fluorosis usually manifests itself as white and gray flecks scattered over the enamel surface. Moderate fluorosis displays dull, unglazed, and sometimes chalky areas over the entire labial and buccal surface and may also display pitting with stain. Severe fluorosis causes pronounced

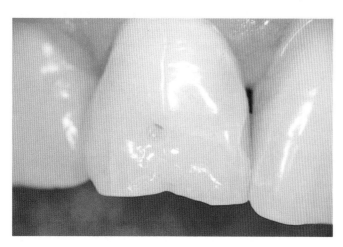

Fig 4-40 Maxillary right central incisor that was deformed during tooth development and is associated with a reduced amount of enamel formation. This is an example of etched enamel, which can take many forms. The effect this irregularity has on the dentin depends on how severely the enamel was affected during its formation.

tooth deformity with abnormal shapes, along with severe pitting stain. Enamel opacity caused by fluoride ingestion is usually poorly demarcated, whereas nonfluoride opacity is well demarcated.

Methods for duplicating mottled enamel (fluorosis) vary with the severity of the case. Mild forms of fluorosis can be duplicated by distributing flecks of gray and white stain after the dentin buildup. These areas of stain should be placed directly on the dentin surface, then covered over with enamel porcelain. Stains are used instead of modifiers because of the strength and opacity needed for duplicating this irregularity. The enamel porcelain covering will contribute depth and subtlety. Moderate and severe cases, however, need more strength and definition; they require gray, white, and any other color found in the natural dentition and are embedded directly into the enamel porcelain, which brings these imperfections to the surface with more pronouncement.

The same procedure is used to obtain this irregularity in all eight methods for duplicating CTC.

Etched Enamel (Fig 4-40)

Etched enamel (hypoplasia) is associated with a reduced amount of enamel formation unrelated to the calcification process. The condition in its mildest state takes the form of horizontal grooves or waves on the labial surface of affected teeth. As the condition progresses, the grooves deepen and eventually expose the dentin, resulting in pitting and discoloration.

Systemic diseases that occur during tooth development usually cause this irregularity and affect the incisors, canines, and first molars more often than the other dentition. In severe cases, hypoplastic teeth may be severely deformed. The region of the teeth affected are the incisal and middle thirds of the central incisors, the incisal third of the lateral incisors, the tips of the canines and the occlusal third of the first molars.

Causes other than systemic diseases during tooth development are trauma, infection, and heredity.

Duplicating this irregularity entails combining surface texture with coloration. In most cases, the needed color can be deep stained into the dentin just at the dentinoenamel junction. The needed grooving (texturing) placed in the enamel porcelain will permit more color to be visible in the thinnest areas of enamel (groove depths). The texturing will regulate the color concentration and location. It is essential to coordinate needed color and texture in order to duplicate this irregularity.

Amalgam Influence (Fig 4-41)

Before fabricating a restoration that will be seated next to an amalgam-filled tooth, it should be discussed with the patient how amalgam affects CTC and whether he or she wants to include this in the ceramic restoration.

The discoloration varies from a very subtle gray, derived from the amalgam, to a dark gray, to black — caused by the corrosion of tin found in the amalgam, which diffuses as metal ions into the dentin. These ions are liberated under the influence of galvanic currents within the restoration and sulfides that presumably originate from saliva.

In cases of extensive discoloration caused by this metal ion diffusion, the patient may prefer to replace the amalgam with a full-coverage restoration in conjunction with the original treatment plan. In most cases, it will be necessary to incorporate at least some of the amalgam influence into the restoration and usually requires a compromise. To completely ignore its effect could cause the restoration to stand out, contributing to its artificiality. A good rule to follow is to routinely lower the value of the restoration to any degree necessary to blend the restoration with the adjacent amalgam-filled tooth.

When incorporating the amalgam influence into a ceramic restoration, it must be pointed out that even though the amalgam restoration gives the impression that the tooth is very dark and low in value, if the amalgam were to be removed, the tooth's appearance would be quite different; in fact, the value will have been raised greatly, revealing four distinct color dimensions. Therefore, when fabricating a ceramic restoration next to an amalgam restoration, the four color dimensions should be accurately detected and measured, using the value dimension (enamel porcelain) to regulate the amount to gray necessary to exactly duplicate the amalgam effect. A common mistake is to attempt to regulate the value by adding gray to the dentin. This violates the hue-chroma and maverick dimension and alters their effect in pro-

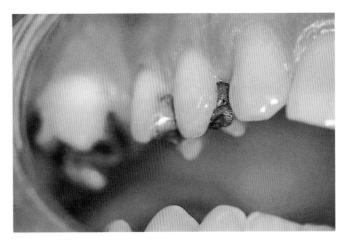

Fig 4-41 Maxillary right posterior quadrant showing the effect amalgam has on CTC. Note how the value is lowered in the premolars and molar as compared to the canine. When restoring a tooth next to an amalgam restoration, the question often arises whether the restoration should comply with the lower value produced by the amalgam, or whether it should maintain the same value as the remaining dentition. In most cases, the restoration should be slightly lower in value so as to blend with the amalgam. A small amount of gray modifier is added to the enamel porcelain.

ducing accurate CTC. The fact that enamel covers the crown of the tooth completely should make it logical to cover the restoration completely with enamel porcelain, thus affording the ceramist an opportunity to duplicate the amalgam influence by regulating the amount of gray added to the enamel porcelain while maintaining the three remaining unaltered color dimensions.

The procedure is the same in all eight methods for duplicating CTC; the entire responsibility for regulating the amalgam influence (lowering value) is placed on the enamel porcelain by adding the proper amount of gray modifier. In most cases, it is not advisable to duplicate the exact value dimension; rather just approach it with slightly higher value to create a better blend with the teeth in the entire quadrant.

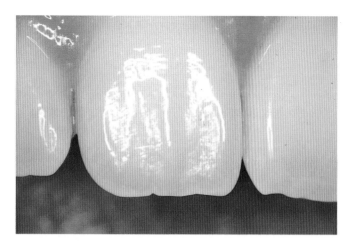

Fig 4-42a Maxillary right central incisor with a high degree of texture typical of young people. Restorations for most young patients require some degree of texture. A more naturally textured surface can be created when incorporated in the enamel during porcelain buildup. This is accomplished with a series of brushes with bristles of different lengths. It is more difficult to obtain a natural texture in the fired porcelain; however, it can be done with diamonds and stones.

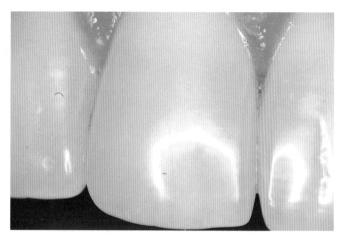

Fig 4-42b Maxillary right central incisor with no visible texture. This texture could be considered a satin texture and is best achieved after firing by using a series of stones and wheels, progressing from a stone with very fine grit to a silicone wheel with much finer grit to a white rubber wheel with no grit. This will develop a satin texture with only a slight glaze. When more glaze is needed, a tin oxide wheel, diamond paste, and zerium oxide with alcohol can establish any desired glaze.

Texture and Glaze (Figs 4-42 to 4-44)

Texture and glaze are so closely related it is difficult to refer to one and not the other. Even though the final texture and glaze of the restoration are just as important as the composite tooth color, they are often overlooked and their importance, underrated. The restoration, whether it be a single unit or a full maxillary or mandibular arch, may be fabricated to perfection, but if the texture and glaze are not duplicated precisely, the finished product could be unacceptable. Only under extreme circumstances could texture and glaze, or lack of either, be referred to as an irregularity; however, there are degrees of each and they vary greatly from mouth to mouth.

Texture

Texture is created during enamel formation and tooth development. A degree of texture is usually found in young teeth. With age and wear, this texture often disappears, giving way to a smooth, dull surface. Texture, or lack of it, has little to do with the health of the tooth. More important is the ability of the enamel to protect the underlying dentin. Wearing away of the texture does not interfere with the enamels' protective quality.

The restoration should include the same amount of texture found in the natural dentition of the patient. Communicating this information to the laboratory can be written or in the form of sample porcelain tabs. The tabs are a set of five, each

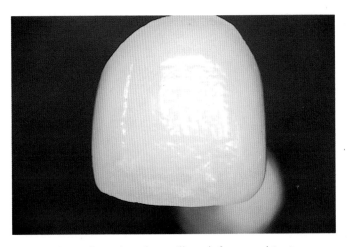

Fig 4-43a Completed maxillary left central incisor restoration that needed texture and glaze. Texture was placed into semiwet enamel porcelain with a texturing brush before firing. To retain the texture and develop prescribed glaze, a hand polishing system was used. (Note subtle hypocalcification spots on the incisal third. They were achieved by applying white stain to the dentin porcelain and covered over with enamel.)

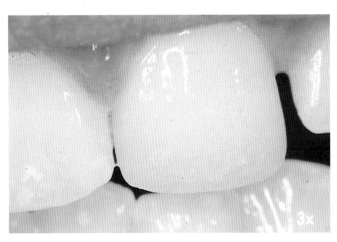

Fig 4-43b Seated maxillary left central incisor restoration. Textured restorations tend to be more lifelike because the saliva that settles over the texture diffuses light in much the same manner as tooth enamel. Therefore, when restoring a full maxillary and mandibular arch, some degree of texture should be included in the restoration.

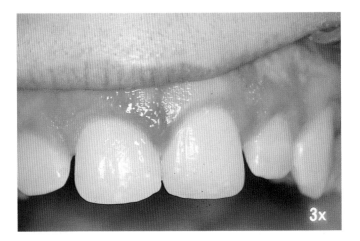

Fig 4-43c Left central incisor restoration compared to natural right central incisor: same texture and glaze. Effort should be made in all restorations to copy exact texture and glaze found on the surrounding dentition.

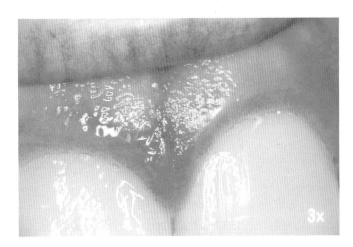

Fig 4-43d Magnified view of left central incisor restoration showing how well the tissue adapts to a well-glazed porcelain margin. Regardless how much texture is incorporated into the restoration, the area beneath the gingiva must be highly glazed with *no* texture. Texture in this area could cause irritation and create an ideal environment for bacterial growth and plaque formation, which could eventually lead to periodontal problems.

having a certain degree of texture and being numbered 1 to 5, no. 1 having no texture, gradually increasing to no. 5, with heavy texture. The ceramist must have an identical set of texture tabs so that when a certain one is prescribed by the dentist the restoration can be textured to that degree.

Surface texture can be derived during two stages of fabrication, pre-and postfiring. To obtain the most natural texture, brushing prefired porcelain is recommended. Brushes with several difference bristle lengths will give the ceramist a choice. The enamel porcelain should be in a semi-wet state during the brushing procedure. With texture brushing, little or no grinding is necessary after firing; accurate contouring must take place during body buildup. If there is a need for postfiring texturing, dull inverted diamond cones work well.

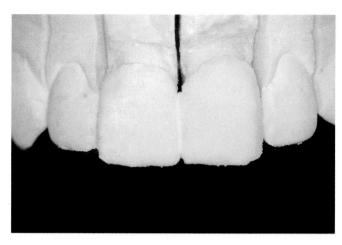

Fig 4-44a Enamel porcelain covering two maxillary central incisor restorations that will have no surface texture. Crowns are built to the needed labial thickness with slight increase in length to compensate for shrinkage. Porcelain surface should be made as smooth as possible in the unfired state.

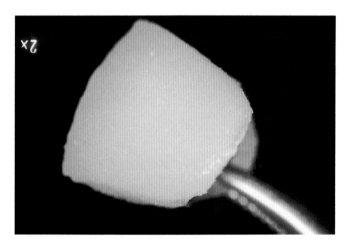

Fig 4-44b Fired restoration, relatively free of labial surface texture. Beginning with a fine stone and progressing from wheel to wheel with finer grits, this restoration will be polished to needed glaze with no texture.

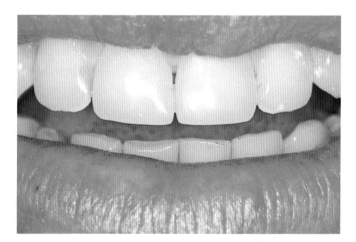

Fig 4-44c Seated maxillary central incisor restorations compare well with the lateral incisors, showing no texture and a satin glaze. Just a slight texture on the labial surfaces of the two restorations could make them unacceptable because of the disharmony they would create with the surrounding dentition.

Glaze

Proper glaze like texture, is an essential ingredient for an acceptable restoration and should resemble that of the other natural dentition. Five sample tabs with varying degrees of glaze can be used to communicate from the dentist to the laboratory. The tabs are numbered from 1 to 5, with tab no. 1 having no glaze while no. 5 is highly glazed. The dentist selects the tab that best resembles the glaze of the teeth surrounding the restoration.

Although in-furnace glazing is the most common method for obtaining a glaze, hand polishing is highly recommended for more control. Hand polishing is especially useful when attempting to preserve delicate subtle texture that would otherwise be lost during furnace glazing.

Furnace glaze. When furnace glazing is used, it is the final firing of the restoration. All functional and esthetic contouring should be completed before this stage because any major adjustment after glazing could require an additional firing, which might prove damaging to the porcelain. If further adjustment is required, consider hand polishing the adjusted areas.

During furnace glazing, the manufacturer's recommendations should be followed as to time and temperature, otherwise permanent damage of the restoration may occur. A surface glaze coating should never be considered when glazing a restoration; the maturing temperature should be reached, giving the porcelain a natural glaze. Surface (super glaze) should not be used for the following reasons: (1) it establishes a specular light reflection as opposed to a diffused light reflection; (2) it contains microscopic porosity, which is an unhealthy environment to the gingival tissue; (3) it tends to nullify delicate labial texture; and (4) it wears away through brushing and mouth acids.

During natural glazing, it might be necessary to withdraw the restoration from the furnace several times for examination before full glaze is reached. Maturing glaze temperatures will vary directly with the amount of color oxides present in the porcelain. Light shades will glaze at a lower temperature than darker shades. For this reason, it is important that the restoration be examined several times before the maturing temperature is reached, to prevent overglazing.

Hand polishing. Hand polishing has several advantages over furnace glazing. Progressing from relatively coarse to finer wheels and pumice and tin oxide, the ceramist has complete control over not only glaze but also, even more important, texture. Hand polishing affords the ceramist the opportunity to select wheels with different grades of grit, using those that will best suit the needs for final texture and glaze. Graduating from coarse stone to high polish, the choices are:

1. Busch Silent Stone
2. Standard silicone wheel
3. Fine silicone wheel
4. Hard rubber wheel
5. Soft rubber wheel
6. Coarse-grit pumice
7. Medium-grit pumice
8. Fine-grit pumice
9. Tin oxide
10. Zerium oxide
11. Diamond polishing paste

Hand polishing is preceeded by a semimature firing (approximately 25°F below full maturing temperature) to completely seal the entire porcelain surface. It can begin from any grit grade and advance to finer grits as needed. There is no set rule in selecting grit fineness; each case will dictate grit requirements.

Hand polishing also saves one firing (glaze firing), which could lead to a stronger porcelain restoration; the less firings, the less chance of complications.

Texture and glaze of a restoration should never be overlooked and must be considered just as important as contour and color. They contribute much to the esthetics of the restoration and should be used to their best advantage.

Summary

Only after composite tooth color has been definitely determined are irregularities considered. Both must be accurately incorporated into the restoration for it to be acceptable. A deficiency in either could result in disappointment.

Composite tooth color influences the tooth uniformly and usually consists of the same color family found in surrounding dentition. Duplication requires accurate detection and measurement of the four tooth color dimensions.

Dividing the tooth into four sections: root and gingival, middle, and incisal thirds; and full labial surface, helps the dentist recognize the irregularities that must be included in the restoration. The patient should be consulted, however, before a decision is made to incorporate the irregularities into the restoration. Also, a good rule to follow is to stress subtlety with less emphasis on irregularities.

Chapter 5

Porcelain Fracture: Causes, Repair, and Prevention

Of all the restorative materials placed in the mouth, well-glazed porcelain (natural glaze without the use of liquid "super glaze") is the kindest to oral tissue. A properly contoured and glazed porcelain restoration causes virtually no gingival problems. Due to the chemical and physical makeup of porcelain, however, fracture of the material can occur. For this reason, you should be familiar with causes and prevention of porcelain fracture. Knowing the chemical and physical composition of porcelain will help establish a better understanding of why these problems exist.

Chemical and Physical Qualities of Porcelains

Porcelains used today are basically crystalline materials such as feldspar, silica, and alumina fused in a glass matrix. Finely ground powders are fired at high temperatures to produce the glass phase, which is translucent by nature and closely resembles tooth enamel. Porcelains are classified according to their fusing temperatures. Medium- and low-fusing porcelains are most commonly used in dental laboratories and in the fabrication of fixed partial dentures, crowns, inlays, onlays, and veneers. High-fusing porcelains are used almost exclusively in the production of denture teeth.

Fritting

Fritting is the process by which low- and medium-fusing porcelains are obtained by fusing the mixed components at prescribed temperatures and immediately quenching the mass in water, which causes cracking throughout. The product is a frit, which is then ground into fine powder and will eventually be used in fabricating the restoration. The fusing temperature will depend on the porcelain's composition.

Color

Porcelain shades are obtained by adding color frits to the unpigmented porcelain. These pigments are produced by fusing metallic oxides with fine glass and feldspar, then regrinding to a fine powder. Metallic oxides and colors produced include iron oxide—brown, copper oxide—green, titanium oxide—yellowish-brown, and colbalt oxide—blue. Zirconium, titanium, and tin oxide are used to control translucency by introducing degrees of opacity.

Composition

Each component of porcelain serves a certain purpose and must be included in proper proportions so that the final product serves the needs of the restoration.

Feldspar

Feldspar is made up of a mixture of potassium silicate and albite and usually makes up approximately 80% of the composition. Natural feldspars are never pure; they contain a varying ratio of potash to soda. The soda form lowers the fusion temperature of the porcelain, while the potash increases the viscosity of the molten glass. The combination is necessary to maintain ease of manipulation of the porcelain in that it reduces slumping during firing and prevents loss of anatomical form and rounding of margins. The efficiency of the porcelain depends greatly on the quality of the feldspar it contains because it provides a glassy phase that serves as a matrix for a quartz suspension; a poor grade of feldspar could create opacity and hinder lifelikeness.

Quartz

Quartz provides strength to the mixture. At normal firing temperatures it remains unchanged; at high temperatures it tends to stabilize the mass. It makes up between 10% and 20% of the mixture.

Kaolin

Kaolin is a hydrated aluminum silicate and acts as a binder. While its presence in the mixture helps increase molding properties of the unfired porcelain, an overabundance could promote opacity. For this reason, it is present in small amounts (2% to 4%) and in some porcelains is omitted completely.

Glass has a noncrystalline structure and is a poor conductor of heat and electricity. Because of the complex atomic arrangements and strong atomic bonds, dental porcelains are basically inert and use the basic silicon-oxygen network as a glass-forming matrix. Properties such as low-fusing temperature and high viscosity are produced by adding other oxides such as potassium,

sodium, calcium, aluminum, and boric oxides to the glass-forming matrix SiO_4 lattice.

Aluminum oxide generally is used in glass formation to increase hardness and viscosity; boric oxide prevents increases in thermal expansion, which allows an increase in alkali content to lower the firing temperature even further.

Because glass has a noncrystalline arrangement, it is totally nonductile. Movements and slip cannot occur. When it breaks, a brittle fracture results. Compressive strength is high, and theoretically its tensile strength is high. However, because of surface irregularities, the actual tensile strength of a ceramic is relatively low. The shear strength is low because of its lack of ductility. For this reason, care must be taken before, during, and after fabrication of a porcelain restoration. Before: proper mixing (body, modifiers, and stains), powder-liquid ratio, and primary condensing. During: careful application, secondary condensing, proper firing cycle, contour, and glaze. After: care during cementation and equilibration, eliminating any possibility of porcelain fracture.

Types of Porcelain Fracture

Of all the failures associated with restorative dentistry, perhaps if not the most expensive surely the most frustrating is the porcelain fracture. Porcelain is capable of fracture at any time during fabrication in the laboratory, during clinical procedures, or in the patient's mouth. Many fractures can be repaired easily with a relative degree of success, whereas others cannot be repaired quite so easily and with little or no success. The sooner the potential fracture is recognized during fabrication, the easier the problem can be solved with better chance of success. Before an attempt can be made to repair the fracture, an accurate evaluation must be performed in order to determine the cause. Every porcelain fracture can be placed into one of three categories: physical, chemical, and

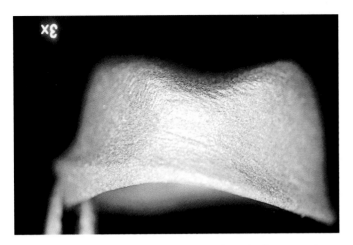

Fig 5-1 Metal substructure must be thick enough to withstand any forces exerted on it. During case planning, it should be determined which alloy will supply the best support with no flexibility.

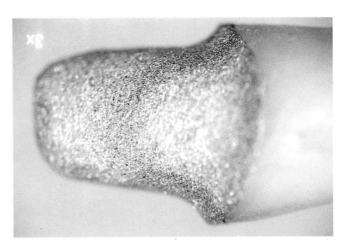

Fig 5-2 The very thin metal margins of anterior castings must be strong enough to withstand flexing during seating, which could cause a porcelain fracture. Physical fractures are repairable, however.

chemophysical. The solution to the problem will depend on this evaluation.

Physical Fracture

Of the three categories, a physical fracture is the easiest to repair with the highest percentage of success. The repair consists of refiring the restoration to its maturing temperature. The cause of the fracture has nothing to do with the chemical makeup of the materials involved. In other words, neither porcelain nor metal substructure has been altered chemically. The cause is a physical antagonist and can be mended with no chemical involvement. The prime concern during the repair is that no chemical change take place that might alter the strength, bonding, or any other requirement for a strong restoration.

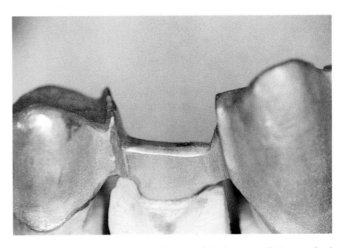

Fig 5-3 In restorations where added strength is needed to withstand excessive load, such as a bar partial removable denture, more metal bulk is required in strategic areas to prevent possible porcelain fracture.

Thin Metal Substructure

The metal substructure must be sufficiently thick to withstand flexing that could cause porcelain fracture or displacement (Figs 5-1 to 5-3). Thickness

requirements vary with the alloy used for the restoration. Under normal conditions, precious alloys should maintain a 0.3-mm thickness throughout, while nonprecious and most semiprecious alloys require a 0.1-mm thickness. Minimum thickness will vary with the location of restoration and

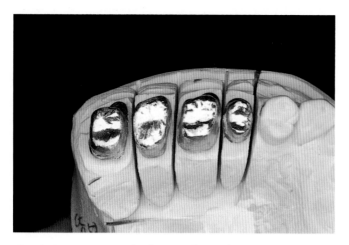

Fig 5-4a Improperly designed metal substructure (lack of interproximal support for porcelain) could result in porcelain fracture. Without support, porcelain could sliver off in this area.

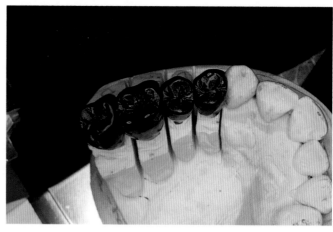

Fig 5-4b A fully waxed version of the restoration will establish ideal occlusion and contour and gives the technician an opportunity to make any necessary functional change in the wax that will eventually be reflected in the porcelain.

functional requirements. For example, in the type of occlusion where the maxillary canines take full responsibility in lateral excursions, a slightly thicker metal substructure should be maintained in this area. Where partial or full group function is used, the extra thickness is not required. Obvious bruxism also calls for extra thickness, as does a case that includes a partial denture in conjunction with a milled substructure. Any splint that will require some manipulation during seating due to nonparallel path of insertion requires extra thickness as well.

When insufficient thickness is the cause of a fracture, the repair can be made easily; refiring at the prescribed maturing temperature will fuse the fracture. Steps should be taken to prevent a reoccurrence of the fracture by repreparing the teeth involved to ensure more ease in seating the restoration, or if need be, by reconstructing the case using proper metal thickness.

Improper Metal Design

An improperly designed substructure is just as dangerous as one that is too thin to support porcelain. The metal substructure must be designed to ensure proper support for the porcelain and thus afford the porcelain optimum strength. A fully waxed version of the restoration will reveal its finished contour. Removing a maximum of 1 mm of wax from the area to be veneered will give the ceramist the opportunity to build porcelain with even thickness throughout, thus assuring the strongest restoration possible. Interproximal areas of single units are often overlooked, and many times unsupported porcelain in this area is prone to fracture. Sharp slivers of porcelain can shear off and become a potential hazard to the patient (Figs 5-4 to 5-7).

In the anterior region, the metal should be designed to eliminate square corners and thin, sharp

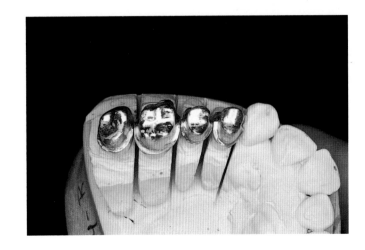

Fig 5-4c A full waxup permits a controlled wax cutback that will ensure an even thickness and provide ideal contour and support for the porcelain. (Note interproximal and occlusal contour.)

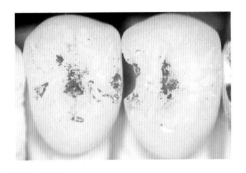

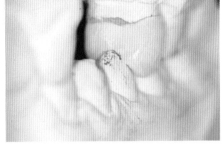

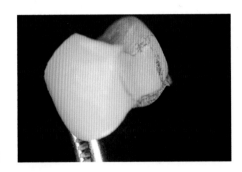

Fig 5-5

Fig 5-6

Fig 5-7

Fig 5-5 A typical interproximal fracture caused by improperly designed metal substructure. If this had occurred in the mouth, complications could have resulted.

Fig 5-6 There are strong opposing forces in the posterior area. Although metal substructure design should vary with needed porcelain support, certain rules are basic, one being interproximal contour that can absorb forces directed there.

Fig 5-7 Fractures such as this require that the substructure be remade with sufficient porcelain support; to simply add porcelain to the fracture area will not ensure a successful repair.

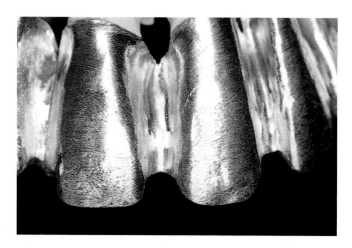

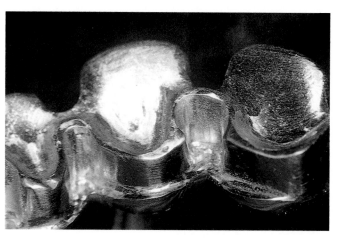

Fig 5-8 Anterior metal substructure should have rounded edges. Sharpness, especially incisally, could develop a cleavage effect, making the porcelain vulnerable to fracture. Line angles and edges should be rounded when dressing and preparing metal for porcelain application.

Fig 5-9 Well-rounded metal contours will lend to a greater compression strength. Carrying the porcelain lingually with no interfering sharpness will help prevent porcelain crazing and shearing. Lingual surfaces should be contoured with a definite ledge at the metal-porcelain junction to make adequate porcelain thickness possible in this area.

edges; cleavage spots could result in a porcelain fracture. Sharp edges reduce the surface area available for porcelain to adhere and thus decrease its compression strength. Well-rounded contours lend to better support, adding more surface area and increasing the compression strength of the porcelain (Figs 5-8 and 5-9).

In the posterior region, the metal design should follow the contour of the cusps to give proper support and prevent shearing when the mandible and maxilla occlude in either centric or eccentric relation. Occlusal forces should be absorbed by the metal substructure (Figs 5-10 to 5-13).

Regardless how strong the metal substructure might be, or its thickness or physical makeup, if it is not designed to give the porcelain proper support, the possibility of fracture is real and case failure could result. Time spent on perfecting metal design saves having to reconstruct the entire restoration.

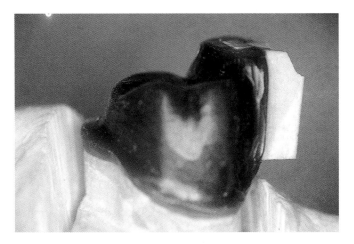

Fig 5-10 In order to obtain maximum function, posterior restorations should be contoured so that the metal substructure absorbs occluding forces. Proper contour begins with a fully waxed restoration, then a cutback that produces ideal occlusal contour.

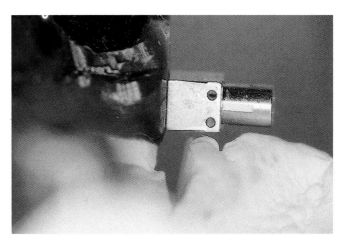

Fig 5-11 The rule for even porcelain thickness (1 mm maximum) holds true, regardless how irregular the contour might be, as when precision attachments are involved.

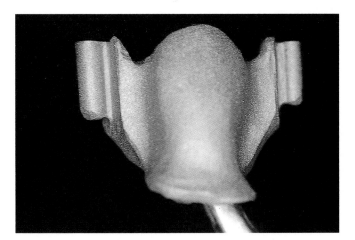

Fig 5-12 Some restorations, such as those that include "dovetails," require other than normal contours. Rounded, well-designed substructures that promote high compression strength are imperative.

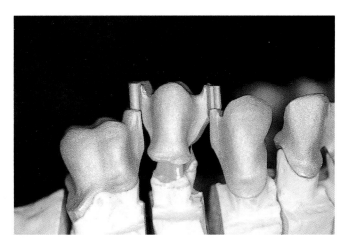

Fig 5-13 In a multiunit restoration, conditions such as occlusal forces and path of insertion must be considered during substructure fabrication. Design should promote ideal function with maximum porcelain strength.

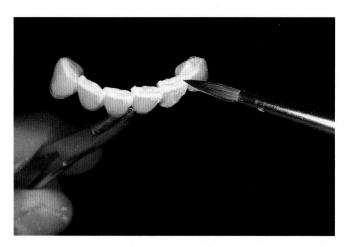

Fig 5-14 Regardless which method is used to apply porcelain, care must be taken not to disturb the porcelain during buildup. A slight separation could go unnoticed and cause weakness, with possible future fracture.

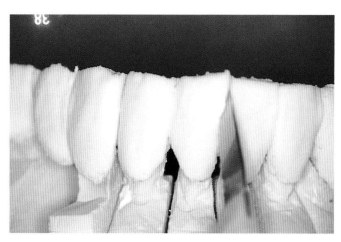

Fig 5-15 It is advisable to slice between units of multiunit restorations before firing; this will ensure equal shrinkage for each unit. If the blade in any way deflects the body porcelain away from the opaque, it could pull away unnoticed during firing, causing a misbond and eventual fracture.

Porcelain Buildup

A porcelain fracture that occurs in the mouth for no apparent reason might have originated during buildup. Any disturbance to the unfired porcelain, whether caused while applying it with a brush or contouring it with a spatula, could create unnoticed separations between porcelain particles and become a weakened area in its fired state. Even the pressure created under vacuum during firing in most cases is not sufficient to push these particles together. In fact, the vacuum may separate them even further when a blade is used to slice between units: take care not to dislodge porcelain either internally or from the opaque layer (Figs 5-14 to 5-16).

Another maneuver during porcelain buildup that could weaken the porcelain to the point of eventual fracture is that of occluding on the articulator while establishing centric stops. Any unnecessary or overzealous manipulation of the porcelain during the buildup stage could dangerously weaken the fired restoration.

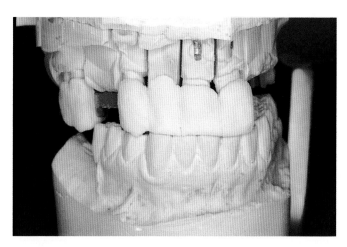

Fig 5-16 Any manipulation of unfired porcelain during body buildup, such as establishing stops and anterior guidance, could dislodge porcelain particles enough to create weakness and possible fracture in the patient's mouth. These particle separations can be so slight that a microscope is necessary for detection.

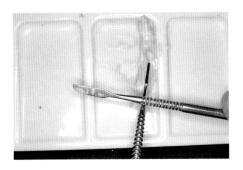

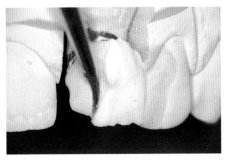

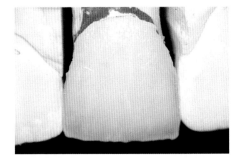

Fig 5-17a

Fig 5-17b

Fig 5-17c

Fig 5-17a Most porcelain should be condensed on the mixing palette before application. This minimizes the necessity for condensing during body buildup, thus lessening the possibility of porcelain slumping and displacement.

Fig 5-17b The need for palette condensing especially holds true in restorations that require delicate placement of internal color characterization. Characterizations should be transferred to the unit in small increments and placed so as not to disturb the previously embedded color. If sufficiently condensed in the palette, just a tap to the master model is enough to establish particle seating and a strong restoration.

Fig 5-17c If porcelain was condensed and applied properly, the fired crown will show undisturbed characterization in prescribed locations with a potentially strong matrix of body porcelain. This unit is now ready for a well-condensed application of enamel porcelain, which should complete a functionally and esthetically acceptable restoration.

Although all porcelains are susceptible to fracture when mishandled during the buildup stage, the fine-grain porcelains seem to be more apt to failure than the coarse grain porcelains.

Inadequate Condensing

The strength of fired porcelain is directly proportional to the amount of condensing. Regardless which technique is used — whipping, vibrating with a serrated instrument, or a mechanical method — a well-condensed porcelain is essential. Thorough condensing should be done on the mixing palette before the porcelain is applied to the metal framework. The porcelain should be in a semiwet state; wet enough so the particles are held together, but not so wet that the mixture flows freely when applied. If the mixture is sufficiently condense before it is transferred to the framework, final condensing is needed only to position it. When color layering is involved, take care not to disturb the layering while condensing (Figs 5-17a to c).

Permitting liquid to remain between porcelain particles during the firing stage weakens the restoration; upon drying, microscopic voids are formed and the porcelain particles are not as closely packed as they would have been had the liquid been removed.

To elimate one cause of porcelain fracture, therefore, consider proper condensing.

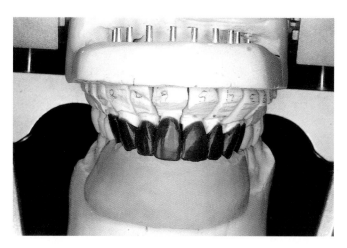

Fig 5-18a Every case should be waxed to full contour. An anterior matrix should be used to designate required length and incisal edge position. This shows you what to expect as to the contour of the completed restoration and also acts as an indicator as to how much wax should be cut back to allow for an even thickness of porcelain.

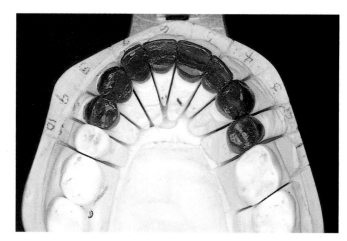

Fig 5-18b A full waxup also enables you to transfer the anterior guidance prescribed for this restoration from the anterior guide table. Once the anterior guidance has been incorporated into the lingual aspect of the waxup, the wax thickness can be measured to determine whether the guidance will be duplicated in metal or porcelain. If the waxed lingual surface is too thin (less than 1.5 mm), the guidance should be duplicated in metal. Otherwise, porcelain would be appropriate.

Porcelain Thickness

Porcelain strength decreases dramatically upon reaching a thickness of 1.5 mm. Its strength relies greatly on compression, which is obtained through the slight built-in coefficient of expansion mismatch between the porcelain and the metal substructure. The compression strength derived from this arrangement is actually the main source. Any other factors, such as proper condensing, vacuum firing, etc, are minor influences in comparison. Porcelain thickness and metal support are related in that improper metal contour could produce uneven porcelain thickness with weakness and eventual fracture.

One way to ensure proper porcelain thickness is to wax the restoration to full contour and cut back 1 mm of wax throughout the entire surface to be veneered (Figs 5-18a to e). This means that the wax that has been removed will represent the thickness of porcelain that will eventually cover the metal substructure. This is a more accurate way to control porcelain thickness and thus maintain maximum porcelain strength over the entire restoration. This method for controlling porcelain thickness is much more reliable than the coping method, in which no effort is made to maintain an even thickness. The coping method is not only guilty of providing a substructure with space for uneven, thick porcelain, it also neglects to provide proper support. This promotes weak, unsupported porcelain that could eventually fracture. For optimum strength based on thickness, porcelain should have a maximum thickness of 1 mm, with sufficient substructure to withstand opposing forces.

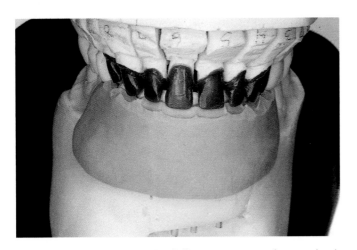

Fig 5-18c Only after the full waxup is satisfactory both functionally and esthetically, should the cutback take place. The wax is gradually cut back and measured for even thickness over the entire surface, using the anterior guide table and index as a standard. The final contour of each unit will indicate the exact amount of porcelain that will eventually be applied to the metal substructure; it should be within 1 mm of thickness and should be distributed uniformly over the entire unit for maximum compression strength.

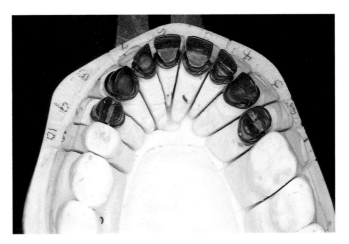

Fig 5-18d If enough thickness is available lingually, the anterior guidance can be registered into the porcelain. However, like other areas of the unit, the porcelain application should be evenly thick and well supported with a properly contoured metal substructure. Because of the tremendous forces directed here, this area must be exceptionally strong and able to absorb these forces with no chance of fracture. A cutback after a full waxup will ensure this.

Forceful Contacts

The stronger the porcelain is, the less apt it will be to fail with any type of forceful contact. Porcelain with proper condensing, thickness, and substructure can usually withstand tremendous forces. However, even the strongest specimen is vulnerable to fracture under certain conditions through accident or otherwise. This could happen either in the laboratory or operatory. Because this is a typical physical fracture, it can be repaired quite easily with no complications or fear of refracture.

Spacing for Postsoldering

In a case involving postsoldering, space between units must be eliminated; by the same token, however, tight contacts could cause porcelain fracture during soldering procedures, due to expansion. The spacing between units need not be wide; light

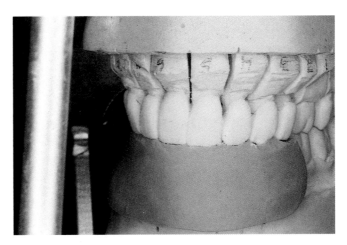

Fig 5-18e The wax cutback from the original full waxup will be replaced with porcelain. With the help of the anterior index, porcelain application is routine and predictable results in that exact uniform thickness will be obtained. Uniform porcelain thickness, therefore, is a prime determinant in preventing porcelain fracture; any violation during this phase of fabrication could result in weakened porcelain that is prone to fracture.

contact is sufficient to prevent a "see-through" connection while allowing enough room for expansion. Although expansion is very slight and in most cases microscopic, a tight contact remains a potential cause of fracture.

Porcelain fracture caused by tight contacts during postsoldering can be readily repaired by refiring; however, several complications are involved. First, the units must be separated. Further, before the fractured unit can be placed into the furnace for refiring, the casting must be perfectly solder free. The area of the crown in direct contact with solder tends to draw some of it into its structure. All of the solder must therefore be removed before refiring the unit, otherwise a black, bubbly crust brought about by temperatures necessary for repairing the porcelain will form. Any solder that soaks into the metal can not only hinder a future soldering effort, but also could cause gassing, resulting in porous porcelain and possible fracture. To be certain this area is completely solder free, the surface should be ground away until all traces of solder have been removed. If this leaves a gap between the crowns that is too wide for soldering to take place, fit a wedge of new alloy into it so solder will flow throughout the connection, uniting the new metal with that of the crowns. This will ensure a strong connection.

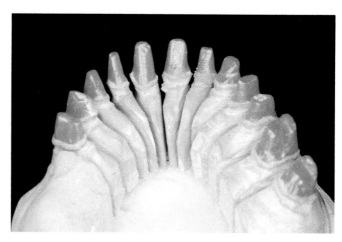

Fig 5-19 During the waxing stage, if there is any difficulty in drawing the wax pattern from the master model, corrections should be made. Undercuts should be filled and the path of insertion changed along with any other needed adjustments. In some cases, the wax pattern will distort just enough to draw away from the die, thus rendering the undercut acceptable, but the casting will prove otherwise. Any change in the master model to eliminate a possible porcelain fracture should be relayed to the dentist so that any needed correction in tooth preparation can be made in the mouth. This could help prevent porcelain fracture during placement. (If fracture occurs before these corrections are made, however, this is considered a physical fracture and can be repaired by refiring.)

Excessive Force During Placement

A single unit or splint may survive the entire laboratory procedure from the waxed version to the finished restoration only to encounter a problem during placement. Even though the restoration may fit the master model perfectly, slight tooth movement could create seating difficulty. Any condition in the mouth that might prevent the restoration from seating perfectly should be corrected *before* an attempt is made to permanently place the restoration. However, if a porcelain fracture occurs during placement due to excessive force, it can be classified as physical and therefore can be repaired by refiring (Fig 5-19).

Chemical Fracture

Although a physical fracture is relatively uncomplicated and simple to repair, a chemical fracture is complicated and impossible to repair permanently. The cause of this type fracture is a chemical imbalance between the porcelain and its metal substructure. A chemical fracture will almost always reoccur regardless of how many attempts are made to repair it. The repair can last anywhere from a day to a few months, but eventually the fracture will return. The chemical imbalance is caused by an abnormally mismatched coefficient of expansion between the porcelain and its metal substructure and usually occurs during casting.

Any procedure during casting that might alter the intended chemical makeup of the alloy could bring about this problem in the coefficient of expansion.

Overheating Alloy During Casting

Manufacturers prescribe definite casting temperatures for each of their alloys. These temperatures depend on the alloy composition that determine coefficient of expansion with a given porcelain. A common cause of chemical fracture is overheating the alloy during casting. Heating the alloy to a temperature higher than that suggested by the manufacturer could burn out any one of several trace elements that regulates the coefficient of expansion, thus creating ideal conditions for a chemical porcelain fracture (Figs 5-20 and 5-21). Although in many laboratories a torch is used for casting, an automatic system such as induction has proven its worth; when properly adjusted, consistent, accurate casting temperatures can be obtained routinely (Fig 5-22). This will help prevent overheating the alloy and maintain chemical balance.

This is not to say that a properly handled torch cannot produce the same results. A well-balanced torch (oxygen and gas), along with the exact prescribed melting temperature of the alloy will produce a complete casting that is free of porosity and chemical change (Fig 5-23).

Therefore, the casting temperature of any alloy used for dental ceramics, regardless which melting technique is used, must be carefully controlled.

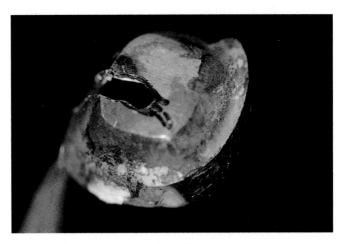

Fig 5-20 Overheating the alloy during casting could deplete needed elements that control the coefficient of expansion and others that control oxidation. Either condition can cause a fracture. Porcelain separates under improper oxidation. Both cases are brought about by a chemical imbalance and are not repairable. Care should be taken to not overheat the alloy; manufacturers' specifications must be observed.

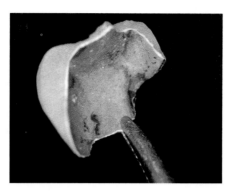

Fig 5-21

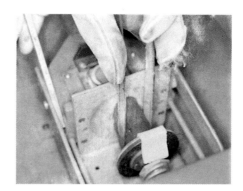

Fig 5-22

Fig 5-21   In order for porcelain to bond to the metal substructure, proper surface oxidation of the metal is essential. Surface oxidation is controlled by the chemical makeup of the alloy. If this chemical makeup is altered, bonding between the metal substructure and porcelain will not occur and a complete porcelain lift-off is possible. In many cases such as this, the entire oxidation layer is removed from the surface of the metal. When this occurs, the metal substructure should be reconstructed.

Fig 5-22   Automatic casting systems can help prevent overheating the alloy. When properly adjusted, accurate casting temperatures will be obtained, thus eliminating the possibility of overheating the alloy, which in turn prevents the possibility of a chemical imbalance. Induction casting has proven to be an asset in many laboratories. Large-volume laboratories should consider an automatic casting system to ensure consistent, accurate casting temperatures.

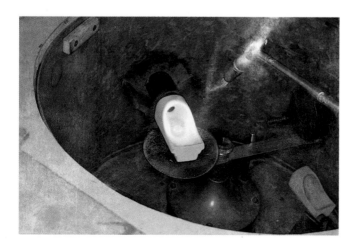

Fig 5-23   When a torch is used to melt an alloy during casting, extra care must be taken to control the melting temperature. Alloys show definite signs when casting temperatures are reached. These signs vary with different alloys and must be recognized. Casting must begin immediately to prevent the possibility of overheating. If the casting temperature is miscalculated, chemical imbalance could result. Therefore, extra care should be taken when using a torch for casting.

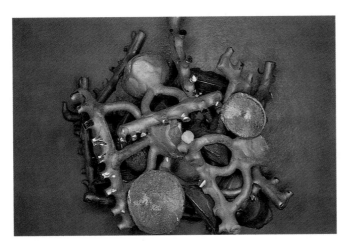

Fig 5-24

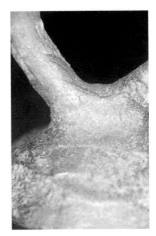

Fig 5-25

Fig 5-24   When adding buttons to a melt, internal and external contaminants might be incorporated into the casting. Any chemical imbalance makes the possibility of coefficient of expansion mismatch greater.

Fig 5-25   Particles of investment, flux, and other contaminants that cling to sprues and buttons often go unnoticed. In some cases, contaminants are trapped internally and are difficult to remove, even when melted. Buttons from precious alloys should be melted and stripped of any foreign materials that might have incorporated internally and externally before they are reused in a future casting. Buttons from base metal alloys should not be reused because the chances for chemical imbalance are greater in base metal alloys than in precious alloys.

Reused Buttons

Most manufacturers condone reusing buttons for casting, recommending using only a certain percentage by weight per ounce of new alloy. In most cases the addition of buttons to a melt will have little effect in the chemical makeup of the casting, but there is a slight chance of chemical imbalance if care is not taken in selecting these buttons. Buttons that were part of a previously abused melt, such as one that was overheated or somehow mistreated so that certain elements were depleted, could contribute to a final casting that lacks the proper coefficient of expansion required for a porcelain bond.

This is especially true in the case of semiprecious and nonprecious alloys. When economically feasible, it is safer to exclude previously cast buttons from the melt. When buttons are used however, they must be cleaned thoroughly to eliminate all clinging investment and other contaminants. In the case of precious alloys, hydrofluoric acid (or a substitute) is used; aluminum oxide blasting is recommended for nonprecious alloys.

A good rule to follow where previously cast buttons are concerned is that if there is a doubt as to their purity and content, they should not be reused; this could help prevent a chemical imbalance and an eventual fracture (Figs 5-24 and 5-25).

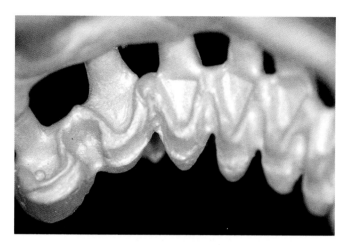

Fig 5-26 Proper waxing, spruing, investing, and casting will ensure a defect-free casting. For multiunit castings, acceptable marginal fits and strong interproximal connections can be predicted. This eliminates the need for presoldering, which could cause several different chemical abnormalities that jeopardize the success of the restoration.

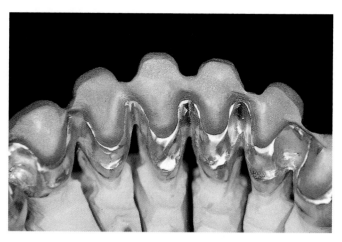

Fig 5-27 The dressed-down multiunit casting, ready for porcelain application, shows strong interproximal connections. Cast connections such as this are advantageous in that (1) they are able to withstand any force directed to them from the opposing arch, (2) they are virtually free of porosity, (3) they consist of the same alloy found throughout the entire casting, eliminating the possibility of internal stress, and (4) the chance of dimensional change during porcelain firing is nil.

Presoldered Connections

A presoldered connection is unnecessary and in many cases could cause problems at almost any stage of porcelain fabrication. With the new and improved materials and techniques available to us, casting multiple units in a single casting can be accomplished with little chance of error, regardless what alloy is used (Fig 5-26 and 5-27). Possible problems are that a soldered connection is not as strong as a cast connection, which could cause porcelain porosity, and warpage could occur during porcelain fabrication. This increases the possibility of a coefficient of expansion mismatch between the solder and porcelain (Fig 5-28).

There are three different alloys in the immediate area of the soldered connection: (1) the mother alloy, (2) solder, and (3) the alloy formed when the solder penetrates the walls of the castings to be joined. This area is often overlooked, especially if the porcelain is not sliced to the opaque layer before each firing. Although it might appear to bond, a microscopic separation could be present due to the distorted coefficient of expansion. The mismatch between the alloy and porcelain covering it might be enough to cause the porcelain to fracture. If the fracture is discovered in the laboratory before delivery, the restoration can be refired to the fusing temperature for repair. Usually the fracture will return, but occasionally it will not and the problem will appear to have been solved. The possibility of future fractures in the mouth is high and, as with all other chemical fractures, chances for repair are remote.

Thermal Rate of Climb and Descent

The difference in thermal conductivity varies between alloys. For this reason, the ideal thermal rate of climb and descent must be selected. To ignore this could mean that the porcelain being processed might remain in any one of the firing stages during maturation either too long or not long enough. The type of alloy and porcelain used in the restoration will dictate the thermal rate of climb and descent (ie, nonprecious alloys should be fired at a rate of approximately 55°F/min; precious, 85° to 100°F/min). To violate this firing schedule could result in either underfired or overfired porcelain, which again could bring about a coefficient of expansion mismatch and a chemical fracture that would be impossible to repair.

Chemophysical Fracture

A chemophysical fracture has a chemical cause but can be treated and repaired like a physical fracture. It is slightly more complicated than a physical fracture but not quite as complicated as one caused by a chemical reaction.

Causes usually associated with a chemophysical fracture are: (1) porous metal substructure, (2) opaque porosity, (3) incorporated contaminants, and (4) interproximal separations and are discussed below.

Porous Metal Substructure

Porosity in the metal substructure is usually located internally; however, occasionally it will appear on the substructured surface. Several conditions can cause a porous metal substructure: (1) improperly sprued wax pattern, (2) improper placement of the wax pattern in the casting ring, (3) improper torch adjustment, (4) insufficient alloy volume, and (5) casting force and venting. Metal porosity can range in size from microscopic to obvious to the naked eye.

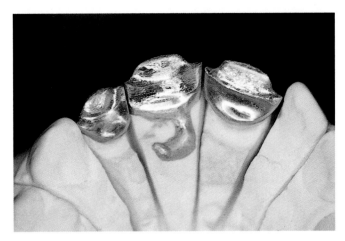

Fig 5-28 Presoldered connections could contribute to a chemical-type fracture due to the potential coefficient of expansion mismatch developed in the interproximal area. Incorporating solder into the restoration introduces a foreign material that differs from the casting alloy. Porcelain bonding in this area could be incomplete, causing weakness and possible fracture. Several porcelain firings can bring about distortion and further add to the problem. For these reasons presoldering should not be considered. A single multiunit casting is preferable.

Improperly sprued wax pattern. The sprue should permit enough alloy to flow so that the cavity is filled with maximum alloy volume before solidification. Generally, it is advisable to fill the cavity with an indirect flow of alloy, graduating from a 8-gauge feeder sprue into a smaller 10-gauge sprue, which eventually flows into the cavity. If the cavity is not filled with the needed maximum volume of alloy, porosity could result.

Improper wax pattern placement. When the wax pattern is positioned in the "thermal zone" (the area in the casting ring where the alloy will solidify last), there is danger that the feeder sprue or reservoir will solidify before the casting, thus depriving the cavity of maximum alloy volume and creating porosity. The wax pattern should be positioned out of the thermal zone, permitting the feeder sprue or reservoir to be located there. It will ensure a continual flow of molten alloy until the cavity is filled to maximum.

Improper torch adjustment. Regardless which casting system is used, correct melting procedure is imperative. In an automatic casting system, most of the variables are controlled. However, when a torch is used to melt the alloy, these variables must be controlled manually.

Improper torch adjustment could be the source of several potential problems. Overheating or underheating the alloy could result in a porous substructure; overheating will burn out needed trace elements, while underheating will cause the molten alloy to solidify before the cavity is filled to its maximum capacity. Porosity will vary from slight in thin veneers to intense in large pontics.

Melting temperatures suggested by the manufacturer should not be violated, and the torch should be regulated so that the correct amount of oxygen is incorporated into the mixture. An excessive oxygen-to-gas ratio could introduce porosity into the casting. Also, natural gas could introduce contaminants into the casting, which in turn could burn during fabrication, giving off gases that form porosity in the porcelain. For this reason, bottled gas is recommended over natural gas.

Insufficient alloy volume. Insufficient alloy will deprive the cavity of needed density to produce a solid casting free from porosity. Enough alloy must be supplied to ensure an adequate reservoir to fill the cavity completely before solidification.

Casting force and venting. The casting force must be enough to push the molten alloy into the cavity while at the same time permit heat and gas to escape. Sufficient force is determined by the amount of needed alloy and its specific gravity. The lower the specific gravity, the greater the force needed to complete the casting. Casting force is regulated by the centrifugal force of the casting machine (number of turns on the casting arm).

Venting can help evacuate heat and gases created by the molten alloy. This permits heat and gases to escape, which would otherwise prevent the molten alloy from filling the cavity completely and free of porosity.

Opaque Porosity (Figs 5-29a to c)

Porosity can originate in the opaque layer. Several possible causes are discussed.

Steam formation. If the casting is placed into the porcelain furnace before the opaque is completely dry, steam could develop from the superheated opaque liquid. Depending on the furnace temperature and the amount of liquid in the mixture, the porosity could range from microscopic to visible. Possibilities are good that the gases trapped there will eventually surface after several firings and cause porosity to form throughout the entire body buildup.

If the porosity is visible, the loose opaque flakes should be removed by blasting with aluminum oxide. A second application of opaque should then be applied to exposed metal and fired.

To prevent steam formation, the opaque should be thoroughly dried before the casting is placed in the furnace.

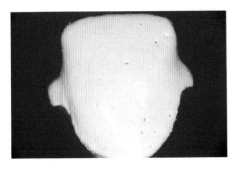

Fig 5-29a

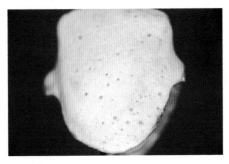

Fig 5-29b

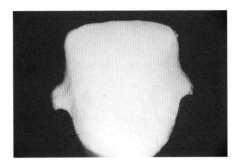

Fig 5-29c

Fig 5-29a   Porosity found in the opaque layer can be caused by indirect and direct factors. It is often difficult to determine the exact cause. However, when opaque porosity is detected, the problem must be corrected before body buildup is begun.

Fig 5-29b   Some types of porosity can be corrected easily; the first step is to clean the surface well by blasting with 50-μm aluminum oxide. This will remove any loose opaque surrounding the porosity while cleansing exposed metal. After rinsing in an ultrasonic cleaner with distilled water for 10 minutes, a thin layer of opaque is applied over the entire casting and fired.

Fig 5-29c   If refiring a thin layer of opaque solves the problem, fabrication of the restoration can continue. If porosity reappears during firing, further steps must be taken to determine the cause. Buildup of body porcelain over porous opaque could cause porosity to form throughout the entire restoration.

Overheating.   Overheating opaque under vacuum could cause porosity (bubbling). Porosity of this type is usually visible. When it occurs under these conditions, it is advisable to completely remove all the opaque and reapply it. Excessively high temperatures, especially with prolonged holding time, could alter the physical and chemical properties of the opaque, thus creating the possibility of inadequate bonding.

Excessive opaque thickness.   A thick application of opaque could prevent the escape of gases that might be expelled from the casting during temperature rise. These gases that are trapped in the opaque may be undetected during this stage and not materialize until as late as the glaze stage. Two separate thin layers of opaque will usually prevent this from happening.

Incorporated Contaminants (Fig 5-30)

Any contaminant that is accidently incorporated into either the opaque or body buildup could cause porosity, which has the potential to surface and cause a void. These contaminants most likely to cause this are those that burn and become gaseous within the firing temperature of porcelain; the gas is formed and expands during firing while seeking an escape. This usually results in a "blow hole" found on the surface of the fired porcelain.

Confining porcelain fabrication to a sealed off, dust-free room will help prevent incorporating contaminants. However, even under the most sterile conditions, one should be on the alert for foreign elements.

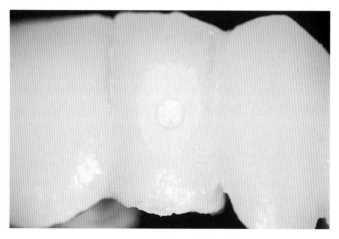

Fig 5-30 When a contaminant becomes incorporated into either the opaque or body porcelain, a "blow hole" could result. This is a typical chemophysical condition. After the chemical reaction is completed (gas formation when contaminant reaches combustion temperature), the repair can be treated like a physical fracture by firing porcelain to the void. Be careful to cover any exposed metal with opaque before adding body porcelain.

Interproximal Separation

Interproximal separation can be visible or hidden and is usually caused by the shrinkage of porcelain toward a more bulky area of the restoration. It could be brought about by interproximal slicing of the porcelain before firing or insufficient opaque bonding at the substructure connections that have been presoldered.

Interproximal slicing. In a multiunit restoration where the units are joined together, if each interproximal area is not sliced during porcelain buildup there is the danger that porcelain in this area will shrink away from the opaque, causing a separation that is often unnoticed and a potential point of fracture. Each unit should be sliced interproximally so that shrinkage is uniform throughout the entire restoration, making each separation visible so more porcelain can be added to fill the void.

Chemophysical Fracture Repair

As previously stated, a chemophysical fracture is not as critical as one categorized as chemical because it can be repaired. In the case of porosity, once the gases have been expelled (chemical reaction), the repair can be performed (physical).

An important step in repairing a fracture of this type is to cover any exposed metal before attempting to replace displaced porcelain. This can usually be accomplished with a combination of opaque and dentin porcelain over which new porcelain is built.

Fractures caused by interproximal separation, such as porosity fractures, can be repaired using the same technique as for a physical fracture. The void caused by porcelain pull-away and shrinkage can be filled and fired.

Summary

Perhaps the most frustrating failure in restorative dentistry is a porcelain fracture. Whether it occurs in the laboratory, operatory, or the patient's mouth, loss of credibility to the technician and dentist could create financial loss and embarrassment.

Some fractures can be repaired easily; others cannot. Only after accurate evaluation can it be determined whether or not the fracture is repairable and a determination made as to how the repair should be carried out.

A physical fracture is rather simple to repair, whereas a chemical fracture is more complicated and, in most cases, impossible to repair. A chemophysical fracture, on the other hand, is slightly more complicated than a physical fracture but not as critical as one where a chemical change has taken place.

Chapter 6

Function, Contour, Color, and Patient Expectations: Case Examples

A properly planned case requires a team effort involving both dentist and technician. Each contributes their expertise to formulate a treatment plan that will not only satisfy the requirements for success but will also live up to the expectations of the patient.

Although function, contour, and color are important in all cases, priority may vary from one case to another. With improvements in preventive dentistry over recent years, caries and periodontal problems are not as prevalent, giving way to more concern for esthetics and cosmetic dentistry.

This chapter presents a series of practical cases, using theories and methods described in previous chapters, to solve various functional and esthetic problems. Some cases are simple and others are more complex; the main purpose is to show, step by step, how these problems can be solved using logical procedures.

Case 1: Fractured Lateral Incisors (Figs 6-1a to i)

Description and Evaluation

A 17-year-old boy fractured his maxillary and mandibular right lateral incisors. The mandibular lateral incisor was eventually bonded, whereas the maxillary incisor showed extensive damage. During case planning it was decided to fabricate a porcelain-to-metal restoration upon completion of endodontic treatment.

Goals and Concerns

1. To restore the look of young vital natural dentition with a porcelain-to-metal restoration.
2. To maintain healthy gingiva with a porcelain margin (platinum foil method).
3. Will use maxillary left lateral incisor as a guide for contour.
4. Will use a customized tooth color (CTC) guide to measure color dimensions in prepared lateral incisor.
5. Duplicating method: no-maverick.
6. Irregularities: (a) white craze lines, (b) slight incisal translucency with dentin frame.
7. Establish ultrafine labial texture with slight glaze.

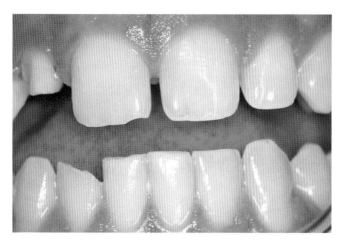

Fig 6-1a Prepared maxillary right lateral incisor (note damaged mandibular lateral incisor). When the prepared maxillary lateral incisor was compared with the unprepared right central incisor during color detection, the composite tooth color (CTC) was obvious, in that the CTC guide matched both precisely. Also, note the absence of maverick color, thus the reason for using the no maverick method for duplicating CTC. Young, healthy gingiva requires special attention throughout treatment, from preparation to final restoration. Maxillary left lateral incisor has dentin frame that extends from mesial to distal and borders the incisal edge. This also must be included in the restoration.

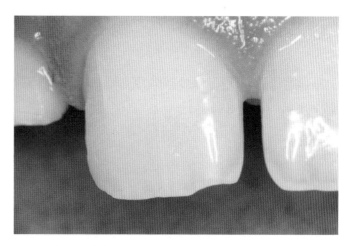

Fig 6-1b Subtle craze lines found in maxillary right central incisor. This irregularity should be incorporated into the restoration to ensure esthetic harmony throughout the maxillary anterior teeth.

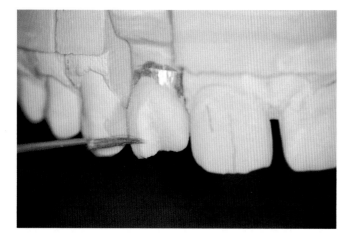

Fig 6-1c When crazing is present in the natural dentition it occurs in the enamel. For subtle results, craze lines are placed into the dentin porcelain during body buildup. This will eventually be covered with a layer of enamel porcelain. A very thin application of white stain is placed over a contoured wall of dentin while layering porcelain vertically from distal to mesial. The stain is mixed with liquid medium. Slight vibration after stain application is required so the medium will unite with distilled water in semiwet dentin. Note platinum foil method for porcelain margin.

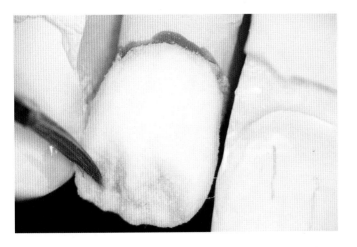

Fig 6-1d A translucent incisal third is included during dentin buildup. A mixture of transparent powder and enamel is placed in the same area as the left lateral incisor. This, in combination with the eventual enamel covering, will give needed translucency in this area. If more transparency is needed, enamel is not included in the mixture; transparent powder is used alone.

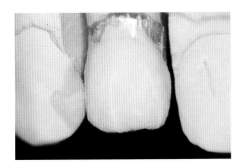

Fig 6-1e

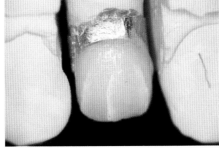

Fig 6-1f

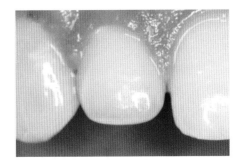

Fig 6-1g

Fig 6-1e Prefired vertical layering of dentin is completed. It is important at this stage to make sure there is enough room for the enamel layer. Areas of overbuilt dentin should be carefully brushed away before buildup is completely dry; this includes mesiodistally as well as labiolingually and incisally. Articulated excursions and protrusive movements at this stage will show functional requirements.

Fig 6-1f Fired dentin buildup revealing craze lines and incisal translucency. Dentin color can be evaluated at this stage with the CTC guide. The selected customized color tab is made up of a layer of opaque covered with dentin. It should match the fired dentin. If there is a color difference, make adjustments before the enamel is applied. The restoration is then contoured and glazed, the platinum is then removed from the margin, and the restoration is ready for seating.

Fig 6-1g Seated maxillary right lateral incisor restoration. Good tissue response at 3-day recall is the result of the porcelain margin. Note the lifelike quality with the very subtle craze lines, the incisal translucency with the dentin frame extending mesiodistally, and the ultrafine labial texture and slight glaze.

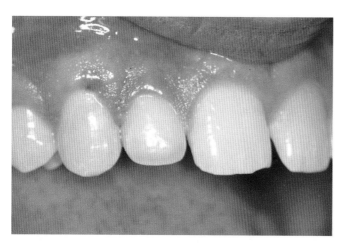

Fig 6-1h The CTC of the restoration blends well with right canine and central incisor. It is common for teeth to vary in color concentration while maintaining the same color family. When restoring six maxillary anterior teeth, it is best to retain the family color while using different concentrations in the canines and lateral and central incisors. This will help contribute to a more natural result.

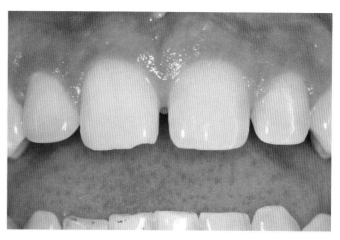

Fig 6-1i Contour of the restored right lateral incisor compares favorably with the left lateral incisor while satisfying all functional needs. Note diastema with slight mesiolabial prominence.

Case 2: Damaged Central Incisors (Figs 6-2a to g)

Description and Evaluation

A 19-year-old man with damaged central incisors as a result of an accident. After endodontic treatment, it was decided to restore the central incisors with porcelain-to-metal.

Goals and Concerns

1. Restoration must be strong enough to withstand athletic endeavors of the patient, thus porcelain-to-metal.
2. Maintain healthy gingiva with porcelain margins (dentin-to-shoulder method).
3. Use 12 anterior teeth for color selection to obtain ideal blend.
4. Duplicating method: maverick plus hue-chroma.
5. Duplicate same basic contour with some minor improvements.
6. Must keep same length and lingual contour for proper function and phonetics.
7. Establish same labial contour and glaze as before tooth preparation.

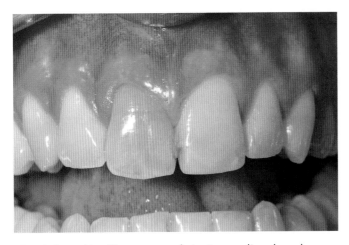

Fig 6-2a Maxillary central incisors discolored as a result of an accident. Right central incisor shows more extensive damage but left central incisor must also be restored. Although function is of most concern in this case, esthetic improvement will also be pursued. The CTC must be selected from unprepared maxillary and mandibular anterior teeth to ensure a well-blending restoration. Maverick plus hue-chroma method for CTC duplication was selected because a thin labial veneer was anticipated.

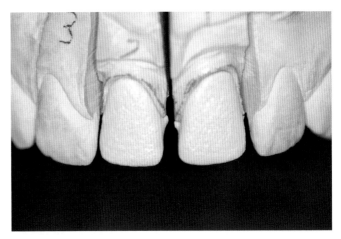

Fig 6-2b Central incisors with transition layer and exposed labial shoulders. Porcelain margins will be incorporated using the dentin-to-shoulder method. Note textured surface of the transition layer for light diffusion. Hue-chroma and maverick color dimensions are included in this layer; the textured surface will transmit these colors back to the eye in a diffused fashion. For a successful tooth color duplication, the CTC should be obtained at this stage. Dentin and enamel covering will contribute to depth and vitality.

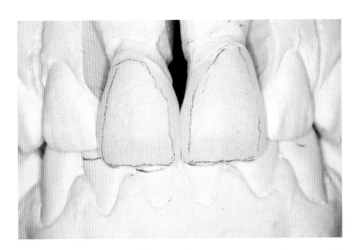

Fig 6-2c Contoured central incisor restorations ready for glaze. Mesial and distal line angles were copied from original diagnostic model with slight change for esthetic reasons. Note steep overbite. Crown length must be duplicated to satisfy function and phonetic requirements. Anterior guide table establishes lingual contour and assists in producing proper length.

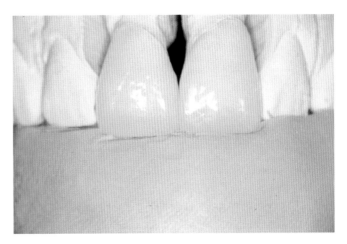

Fig 6-2d Glazed restorations with anterior matrix verifying proper length. Matrix was made from original diagnostic model and is worked in conjunction with the anterior guide table to make certain the crown length is precise. Tissue model was used to give exact location of gingiva in an effort to prevent tissue impingement and/or undercontour. Note slight labial texture and moderate glaze.

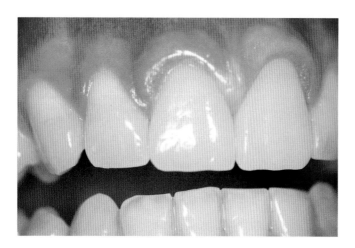

Fig 6-2e Seated maxillary central incisor restorations displaying acceptable CTC that harmonizes with the 12 anterior teeth. Three-day recall shows excellent tissue response to labial porcelain margins. Note worn labial incisal third surface of mandibular anterior teeth. This functional problem dictated a thin labial porcelain veneer on both restorations (approximately 3/4 mm with gold, opaque, transition, dentin, and enamel layers).

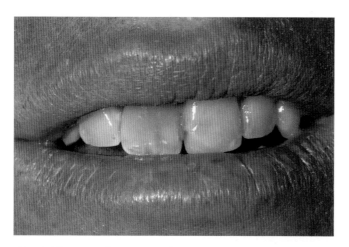

Fig 6-2f Maxillary central incisors before treatment revealing unattractive contour and color. Young patient was self-conscious of his appearance and was concerned as to whether improvements could be made.

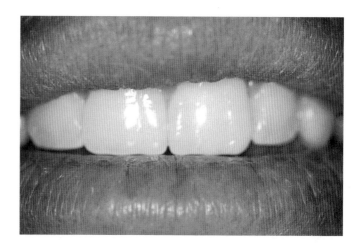

Fig 6-2g Completed maxillary central incisor restoration shows changes in labial contour. A more pleasant smile line was created and esthetics were improved.

Case 3: Devitalized Central Incisor (Figs 6-3a to f)

Description and Evaluation

A 37-year-old man with devitalized maxillary left central incisor. Before preparation, the tooth was slightly twisted, overlapping the right central incisor. Patient preferred that the restoration not overlap and that a more esthetic tooth alignment be established.

Goals and Concerns

1. Restore maxillary left central incisor with porcelain-to-metal.
2. Include porcelain margin to improve gingival health (porcelain margin material).
3. Bring restoration in line with other anterior teeth, but it must be narrower than the right central incisor because of limited space.
4. Must select CTC from left central incisor.
5. Will use maverick plus hue-chroma method for CTC duplication.

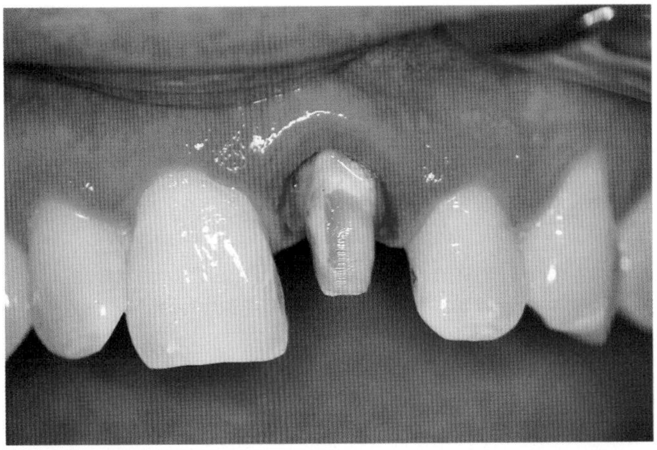

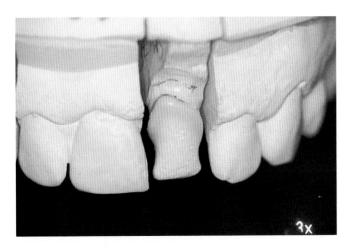

Fig 6-3a Prepared maxillary left central incisor. Discolored dentin made it impossible to use this tooth for CTC selection. Protrusion will greatly limit labial thickness of the restoration where improved tooth alignment is part of the treatment plan, as in this case. Also, the width of the restoration will be narrower than the right central incisor because of original misalignment.

Fig 6-3b Opaqued casting with porcelain margin in place. When using this method for establishing porcelain margins, the material is fired to the casting after the opaque layer has been completed. The reason for this is the difference in the maturing temperature of each material. The maturing temperature of opaque is the highest temperature the porcelain will reach throughout fabrication. The next highest temperature is that of the porcelain margin material (first firing). An addition was made to the margin material to seal the margin completely. This is necessary because of shrinkage of the first application and is fired 5° lower. Note contour of casting needed for porcelain support and fracture prevention.

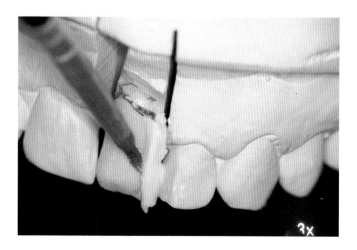

Fig 6-3c Incorporating irregularities (craze lines) during vertical layering of dentin porcelain. After the second firing of porcelain margin material, the resulting margin is tapered and the transition layer is fired over the entire surface (opaque and porcelain margin). The transition layer contained needed color for CTC, incisal translucency, and frame, as well as gingival and interproximal color modification. These accents will project through the dentin and enamel layers of porcelain almost unnoticed, but they are necessary for exact CTC duplication. In comparing the restoration with the right central incisor it is obvious how thin the finished labial surface will be.

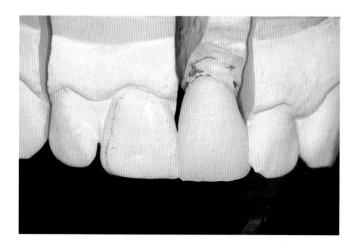

Fig 6-3d Restoration ready for glaze. A thin enamel layer was applied upon completing dentin buildup and both layers were fired together. This can be accomplished in two steps if you are concerned about the resultant dentin firing. Any needed changes can be made before the enamel application. After this firing, the restoration is made functionally sound, is contoured, and is made ready for glazing.

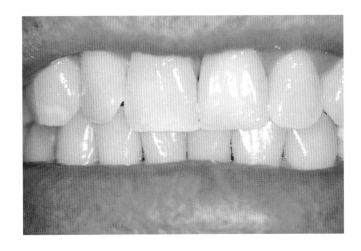

Fig 6-3e Hand polished, seated maxillary left central incisor restoration. Even though labial thickness (metal, opaque, transition layer, dentin, and enamel) measures less than 1 mm, the CTC has been accurately duplicated. An esthetic tooth alignment has been established; however, note how narrow the restoration is as compared to the right central incisor. When proper CTC, contour, texture, glaze, and incorporated irregularities are achieved, often the attention is diverted from a problem such as this, which usually then goes unnoticed.

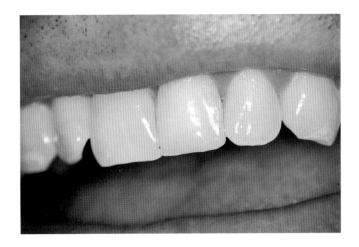

Fig 6-3f Close observation reveals several subtle irregularities that are found in most natural dentitions. Mesial craze lines extend from the gingival to the mid-third of the restoration and correspond to a craze line found in the right central incisor. Also, note interproximal color, incisal translucency, and frame projecting from the transition layer. Transition layers play an important role in every restoration, especially when the labial dimension is very thin.

Case 4: Replacing Extracted Central Incisor (Figs 6-4a to e)

Description and Evaluation

A 25-year-old man with extracted maxillary left central incisor (due to an accident). The patient preferred minimum treatment with the best esthetic results. It was decided that a Maryland bridge would be appropriate with minimum tooth reduction.

Goals and Concerns

1. Replace missing maxillary central incisor with a pontic attached to lingual surfaces of the right central and left lateral incisors (Maryland bridge).
2. Bonding the bridge will be accomplished with a composite resin material (light cured) so that the bridge can be gold plated (acid etching will not permit this).
3. Bridge "wings" must be countersunk to accept light-cured composite resin material.
4. CTC must be selected from maxillary right central incisor.
5. Anterior matrix will be constructed from a waxed pontic. This matrix will be used as a guide for the restoration.

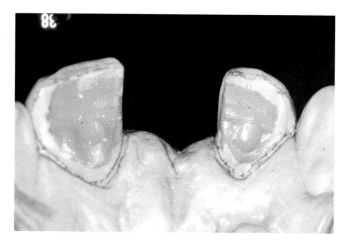

Fig 6-4a Stone master working model for the case. The lingual surfaces of the maxillary right central and left lateral incisors were prepared with minimum tooth reduction. Note interproximal extensions to ensure maximum retention. Sufficient tooth structure must be removed to allow for metal thickness that will be strong enough to support the pontic. Also, the preparation should have a definite finish line so the margins will not bend and/or flake off.

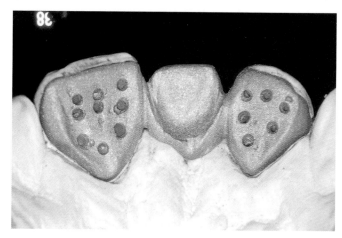

Fig 6-4b Casting with countersunk holes for retention. A tapered carbide bur is used to cut into the casting. The casting should be designed so that none of it shows labially after seating. The preparation must be made so that the casting is just shy of the incisal edge and hidden interproximally with tooth structure. Note pontic design; it must be contoured to give maximum support to the veneer while preventing a food trap at the tissue junction. Metal connections on both sides of the pontic must be strong enough to withstand fracture.

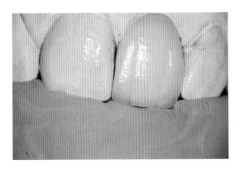

Fig 6-4c

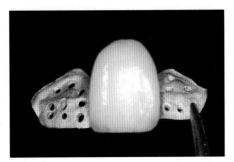

Fig 6-4d

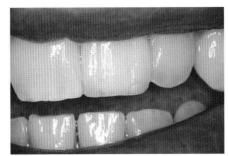

Fig 6-4e

Fig 6-4c Completed Maryland bridge with anterior index that duplicates exact incisal edge position and contour established during waxup. This ensures functional and phonetic needs of the patient.

Fig 6-4d Gold-plated Maryland bridge. When there is concern about metal substructure influencing the CTC of the abutment teeth of a Maryland bridge, gold plating should be considered. The gold-plated "wings" facing the prepared surfaces of the abutments will not lower their value but will help maintain the original CTC. When gold plating is used, the metal cannot be etched for retention.

Fig 6-4e Seated Maryland bridge replacing maxillary left central incisor. Note slight distal overlapping of the pontic, which was necessary to establish the same width as the right central incisor. Also, note the labial surface texture of the pontic and how it compares with the right central incisor.

Case 5: Replacement of Large Amalgam Restoration (Figs 6-5a to j)

Description and Evaluation

A female entertainer with a large amalgam restoration in the maxillary right first molar. The patient was concerned about the noticeable restoration in an otherwise caries-free mouth. It was decided to replace the amalgam with a porcelain-to-metal restoration.

Goals and Concerns

1. The porcelain-to-metal restoration will have full porcelain coverage with no visible metal.
2. Will include porcelain margins using the platinum method.
3. There were no visible color deposits; CTC was uniform.
4. Duplicating method: maverick over opaque.

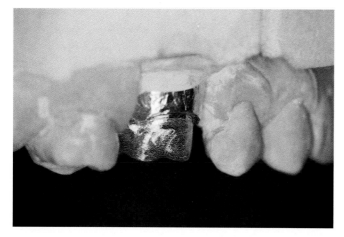

Fig 6-5a Maxillary right molar casting with platinum foil in place over the labial shoulder of the die. Of the three methods for fabricating a porcelain margin, the platinum method is probably the most accurate. The foil is measured, cut, and annealed, then placed over the labial shoulder and burnished. The casting is placed onto the die. The foil should prevent the casting from seating completely on the die labially and lingually.

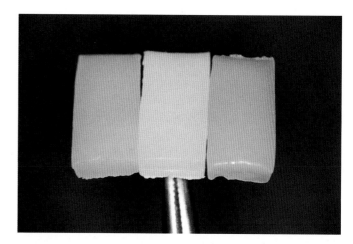

Fig 6-5b Three CTC tabs selected during tooth color dimension detection and measurement. The value tab was selected from the enamel of the tooth, hue-chroma and maverick tabs from the dentin. These tabs will be used as a reference throughout the fabrication of the restoration. If the selections were accurate, CTC duplication should be uncomplicated.

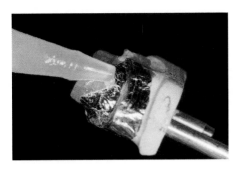

Fig 6-5c

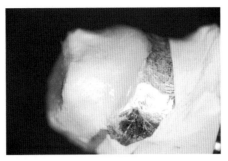

Fig 6-5d

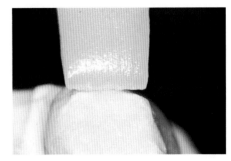

Fig 6-5e

Fig 6-5c   The burnished platinum foil is temporarily attached to the inner surface of the casting with a very small drop of cyanoacrylate. It is held in place while the opaque is fired to it, making it a permanent part of the restoration. Care must be taken to keep the die free of cyanoacrylate so that it will not become attached to the casting.

Fig 6-5d   The porcelain margin is established in a separate firing. Once the platinum is permanently attached to the casting, dentin application begins with the overbuilt shoulder area. Porcelain will shrink toward bulk. The bulky porcelain buildup at the margin will shrink toward the shoulder of the die, thus ensuring a perfect seal. A slight color modification is made at the margin for a a better blend with the margin buildup. All color dimensions are included in this layer. The porcelain margin is ready to be tapered and made ready for the next porcelain application.

Fig 6-5e   Comparing a thin maverick layer with the maverick tab. In the maverick-over-opaque method for duplicating CTC, a thin layer of the selected maverick color is fired over the transition layer. This maverick layer will influence the entire restoration uniformly with no areas of color concentration.

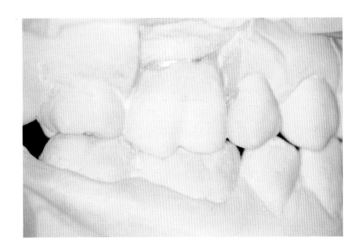

Fig 6-5f   Porcelain buildup ready to be fired. The restoration is built to full contour with dentin and enamel porcelain. Function and contour are incorporated into the unfired porcelain. The more effort made before firing, the less grinding will be necessary after firing. Excessive grinding could remove color needed to comply with the selected CTC. Enamel porcelain is slightly overbuilt occlusally to compensate for shrinkage.

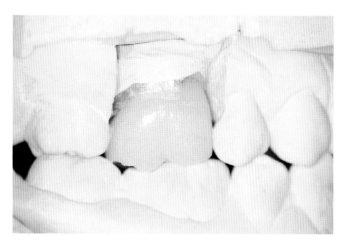

Fig 6-5g The fired restoration placed on the model and articulated. When the restoration is properly contoured during porcelain buildup, only minor adjustment and shaping are necessary. Lateral excursions will dictate occlusal contour while the buccal contour of the remaining natural dentition will dictate the buccal cusp location of the restoration. Special attention must be directed to premature contacts and lateral interferences while maneuvering the articulator.

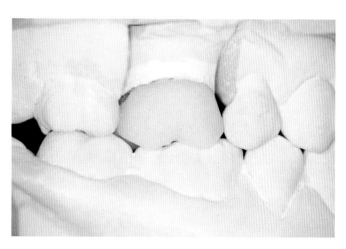

Fig 6-5h Restoration ready to be glazed. After functional and esthetic requirements are fulfilled, the restoration is prepared for glaze. A 25-μm aluminum oxide spray and steam are used to clean the restoration before glazing. The platinum foil must remain in place until after glazing to preserve porcelain margin integrity.

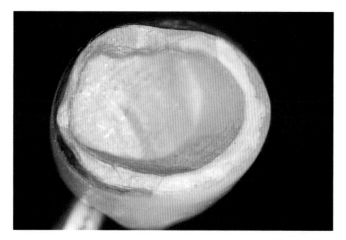

Fig 6-5i Glazed restoration after platinum has been removed is ready for seating. Note the porcelain margin and how the dentin covers the opaque. The platinum foil is attached to the casting with the opaque layer, but enough margin area is left so that dentin will cover it completely. This is important for esthetic reasons and gingival health; opaque is porous and cannot be glazed.

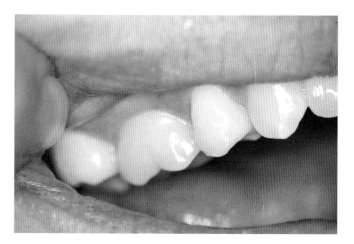

Fig 6-5j Seated maxillary right first molar at 3-day recall. Note tissue response to the well-glazed porcelain margin and absence of visible metal. A metal margin has a tendency to irritate the tissue in this area; even when covered completely with porcelain, it often creates a dark shadow and/or impinges on the tissue. Also note how well the CTC harmonizes with the surrounding dentition by using the maverick-over-opaque method for duplication (an even influence of the maverick dimension throughout the entire restoration with no area of color concentration).

Case 6: Restoration of Central Incisor (Figs 6-6a to p)

Description and Evaluation

A 40-year-old woman with poor oral hygiene habits in need of a restoration for her maxillary left central incisor.

Goals and Concerns

1. Restore maxillary left central incisor with porcelain-to-metal.
2. Include porcelain margin to improve tissue health.
3. Improve function between restoration and mandibular anterior teeth.

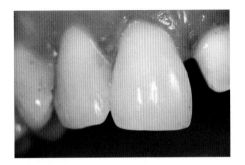

Fig 6-6a

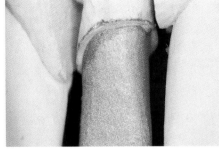

Fig 6-6b

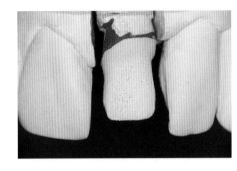

Fig 6-6c

Fig 6-6a Prepared maxillary left central incisor. Note poor oral hygiene, especially the deteriorated condition of the gingiva. A functional problem was the main reason for a restoration.

Fig 6-6b Casting and working die. Note how the casting is contoured to give proper support for porcelain so that maximum compression strength can be obtained. Also, note the ideal shoulder preparation (90-degree angle) for a porcelain margin. Any angle other than 90 degrees in this area makes it difficult, and in some cases impossible, to achieve a perfect marginal seal.

Fig 6-6c Opaqued casting with tapered porcelain margin. Margin area should be contoured to permit enough room for the transition layer. This helps establish the CTC in the gingival area while eliminating opacity.

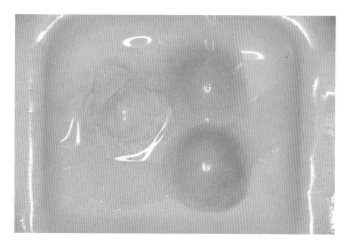

Fig 6-6d

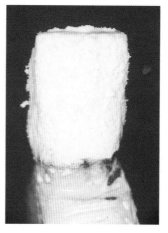

Fig 6-6e

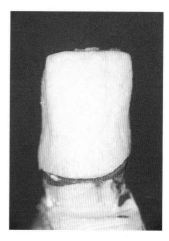

Fig 6-6f

Fig 6-6d Porcelain selection that will be mixed and applied as the transition layer. Composite tooth color is incorporated into this layer and projected through the dentin and enamel porcelain. It creates color depth while diminishing the effect opaque has on the restoration.

Fig 6-6e Prefired transition layer. The transition layer is applied over the entire surface of the opaque. A short, stiff-bristled brush is used to roughen the surface before firing. The rough surface diffuses light as it enters the restoration while transmitting the colors that make it up.

Fig 6-6f Fired transition layer. Maturing temperatures are progressively reduced from the opaque through the transition layer. The maturing temperature of opaque is the highest of the three. Margin porcelain is fired approximately 15° below that of opaque. The second margin firing, which is usually required to compensate for shrinkage, is fired 5° lower than the first firing. Next, the transition layer is fired 10° below the second margin firing and approximately 15° higher than dentin. Note color and texture of fired transition layer. All colors needed for CTC should be recognized at this stage. If necessary, the color can be altered in the dentin application.

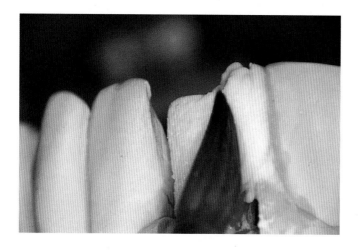

Fig 6-6g Lateral layering of dentin porcelain. As the dentin porcelain is applied laterally from mesial to distal, irregularities are incorporated with stains and body modifiers. Internal characterization is much more effective than external staining. Internal staining must be done in moderation, because excessive color oxides could alter the coefficient of expansion of the porcelain and cause a fracture. When stain liquid medium is used, slight vibration is necessary to mix the liquid with distilled water in the dentin.

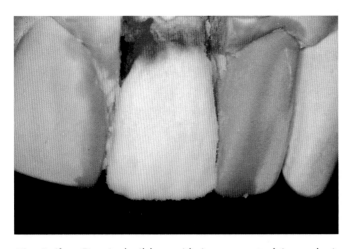

Fig 6-6h Dentin buildup with incorporated irregularities. Before the restoration is fired, functional and contour requirements must be evaluated. The anterior index will determine proper length and labial thickness, allowing enough room for enamel porcelain. Enamel can be applied either at this stage or after the dentin firing. If there is concern with the fired dentin, enamel porcelain should be fired separately, allowing for any needed alterations in the dentin.

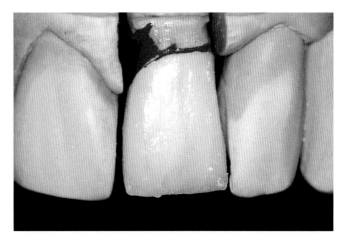

Fig 6-6i Fired dentin application. Note subtle internal characterization (several check and craze lines) along with incisal translucency and color dimensions needed for the restoration's CTC. Although in natural dentition these irregularities are located in the enamel, when placed in the dentin of the restoration, results are more natural looking. When there is limited space for porcelain, as in restorations such as this, the enamel layer will be very thin. It is difficult to include these irregularities in an enamel layer this thin. Note slight opening at labial porcelain margin brought about by shrinkage. This will be resealed during the glaze firing.

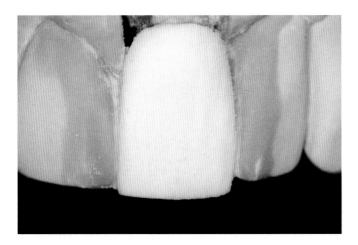

Fig 6-6j Prefired enamel porcelain application overextended incisally to compensate for shrinkage. It covers the dentin completely, and although thin, it is necessary to satisfy the value dimension. Underlying color dimensions and irregularities will easily project through.

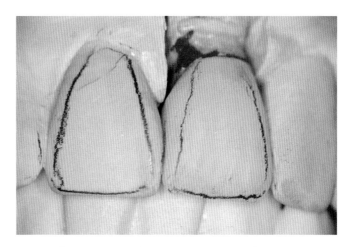

Fig 6-6k Contoured restoration ready for glaze. Line angle location and general contour are copied from the right central incisor. Labial texture should also be noted before glaze. Functional requirements must also be met at this time (ie, lateral excursions, protrusive movement, and centric stops).

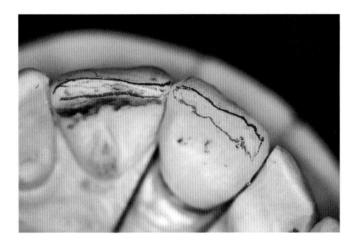

Fig 6-6l Lingual and incisal views of restoration. The incisal edge position and contour were established through lateral excursion and protrusive movements, whereas the lingual contour was established with the anterior guide table. Note centric stops on lingual surface; they are necessary for stabilization and to prevent the tooth from extruding.

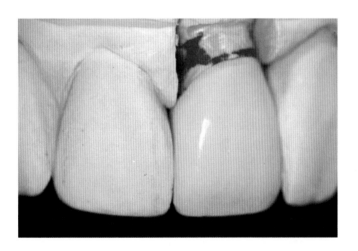

Fig 6-6m Glazed restoration on model, ready to be seated. Glazing can be accomplished by firing or hand polishing. In this case, firing was required because of the needed marginal seal due to shrinkage (see Fig 6-6i). Occasionally, the dentin firing will pull the margin material away from the shoulder. When this occurs, a mixture of dentin and margin material (3:1) is applied to the margin and fired, under vacuum, during the glaze bake.

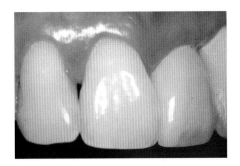

Fig 6-6n

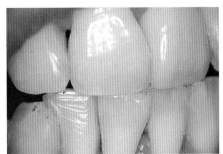

Fig 6-6o

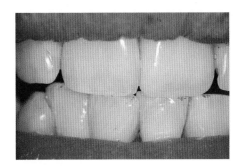

Fig 6-6p

Fig 6-6n Seated maxillary left central incisor at 3-day patient recall. Note how well the tissue has adapted to the porcelain margin and the overall improvement in oral health (see Fig 6-6a). When an addition is made to the porcelain margin during the glaze bake, it is necessary to hand polish this area to a high glaze before seating.

Fig 6-6o No adjustments are needed during left lateral excursion. If the restoration is properly manipulated on the articulator, little if any adjustments are necessary after seating. Although the restoration measures less than 1 mm labially with metal, opaque, transition, dentin, and enamel layers, the CTC blends well with the right central incisor. Also, note the same degree of texture and glaze.

Fig 6-6p Protrusive movement. The anterior guide table of the semiadjustable articulator is responsible for minimizing the need for incisal and lingual adjustments. For a restoration, whether it be a single unit or a full arch, to be an ultimate success, the technician must make certain that every functional need is satisfied before the case is delivered to the dentist. The more adjustments necessary at the chair, the less chance the restoration has of surviving. It could cause porcelain weakness with loss of color and contour.

Case 7: Restorations Causing Gingival Irritation (Figs 6-7a to v)

Description and Evaluation

A 30-year-old man with two restorations (maxillary right central and lateral incisors). The patient was concerned with the gingival reaction to the restorations. Preliminary evaluation during case planning revealed well-sealed, functionally sound restorations. Further observation revealed undercontouring of the gingival area with exposed metal margins that caused tissue irritation.

Goals and Concerns

1. Restore maxillary right central and lateral incisors and improve color and contour.
2. Include porcelain margins in restorations (dentin-to-shoulder method).
3. Use tissue model to establish tissue location.
4. No maverick duplicating method will be used to develop CTC.

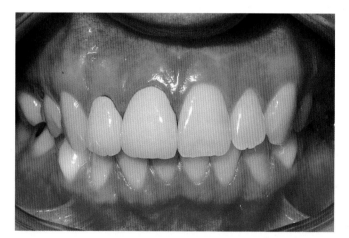

Fig 6-7a Preoperative condition. Maxillary right central and lateral incisors are undercontoured at the gingival third. Note metal collar exposure, which has caused tissue irritation in this area. Although the restorations are functionally sound with satisfactory seal, they are unnatural looking due to lack of porcelain vitality and proper CTC duplication.

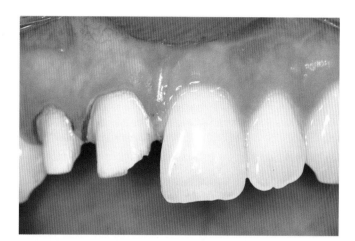

Fig 6-7b Prepared maxillary right central and lateral incisors. Note absence of maverick color in dentin, which dictates the CTC duplicating method of no maverick. Compare dentin of prepared right incisor with unprepared left incisors. The CTC is easily recognized, and a CTC guide could be used with any of the four. In most cases where unprepared teeth must be used for detecting and measuring tooth color dimensions, a CTC guide is quite accurate.

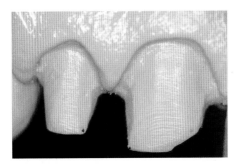

Fig 6-7c

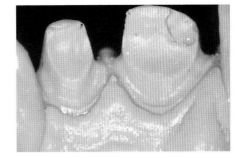

Fig 6-7d

Fig 6-7c   Labial view of the tissue model that will be used to help contour the restorations in this area. Overcontouring could impinge on the tissue, whereas undercontouring could create spaces between the teeth that often cause esthetic and phonetic problems.

Fig 6-7d   Lingual view of tissue model. The lingual surface of the tissue model will dictate the lingual contour of the metal substructure of the restorations. The wax patterns are transferred back and forth from the working master model to the tissue model until they satisfy all the lingual requirements. Lingual contour must begin during the waxing stage because it is difficult (and in some cases impossible) to change a miscontoured metal casting.

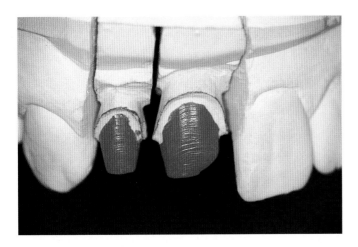

Fig 6-7e   Dies of the working master model are coated with a spacer material before waxing. The spacer provides space for cement during seating. The material is a very thin lacquer and is applied in several layers, depending on the amount of space needed. On a full-arch multiunit restoration, more space should be provided to allow tolerance for seating. It is never carried over the labial or lingual margins; leakage would result.

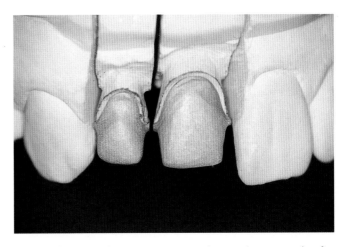

Fig 6-7f   Metal castings seated on dies, ready for opaque. Patterns can be waxed either shy of the labial shoulder or on to the shoulder, and the metal can be cut back after casting to accommodate porcelain. Note design of metal substructure for maximum porcelain support. Before opaque application, the castings are blasted with 50 μm of aluminum oxide then steam cleaned.

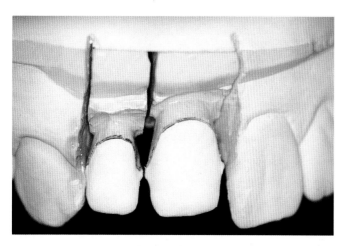

Fig 6-7g Transition layer. The transition layer was applied over the opaque layer (separate firings at different maturing temperatures) and extended to the shoulder of the die. Composite tooth color is incorporated into this layer and is evident upon firing.

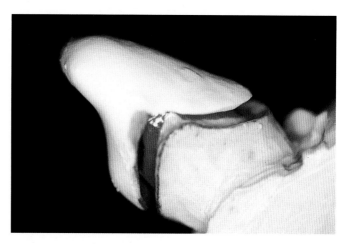

Fig 6-7h Well-condensed transition layer in the margin area. The transition porcelain should be vibrated to ensure a well-condensed porcelain margin. Shrinkage in this area is inversely proportional to how close the porcelain particles are placed. In spite of the condensing, slight shrinkage will occur. This will be compensated for during the glaze firing.

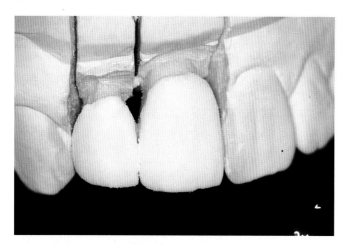

Fig 6-7i Prefired dentin application. The dentin layer is applied after the transition layer has been fired. A 1:1 mixture of transition porcelain and dentin is placed in the area of shrinkage before the dentin application, which is extended to the shoulder of the die. This can be fired separately or together with enamel porcelain.

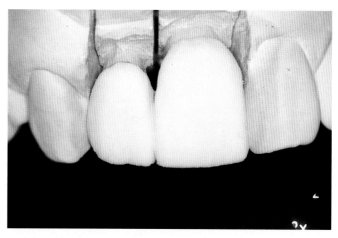

Fig 6-7j Prefired enamel layer. A thin layer of enamel porcelain is applied over the entire restoration to satisfy the value dimension. In cases such as this, where the maverick dimension is not involved and colors are uncomplicated, dentin and enamel layers can be fired together with predictable results. This is especially true when the CTC is verified during the transition stage. The enamel layer is slightly overextended incisally to compensate for shrinkage.

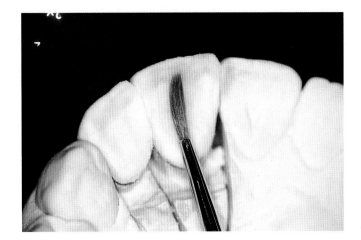

Fig 6-7k Staining prefired enamel porcelain. Needed color modification should be made with modifiers and stains internally or externally before firing. When subtle incisal color is needed, a thin application of stain is placed lingually so that its effect will be transmitted labially in a natural, lifelike manner. The color family and intensity should be recognized during CTC detection.

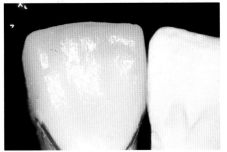

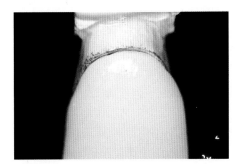

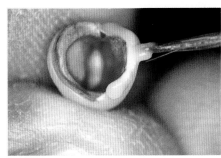

Fig 6-7l

Fig 6-7m

Fig 6-7n

Fig 6-7l Fired enamel porcelain with obvious results from linguoincisal stain application to prefired porcelain. Incorporating color to unfired porcelain is preferred to surface staining postfired porcelain because of the more natural results. Note how the stain has mildly penetrated the porcelain. The color will remain during the life of the restoration, whereas a surface stain will eventually disappear with wear and mouth acids.

Fig 6-7m Fired dentin and enamel revealing labial porcelain margin shrinkage. Shrinkage is anticipated when using this method to obtain a porcelain margin. The margin can be reestablished either by adding in a separate firing or during the final glaze bake. In this case, the addition will be made in a separate firing, after which hand polishing will be used to develop a glaze.

Fig 6-7n Resealing the porcelain margin. A 1:1 mixture of stain liquid medium and distilled water is added to a mixture of dentin and transition material and spatulated to a doughlike consistency. This substance is then applied to the entire labial margin. The glycerine in the stain liquid medium helps keep the mixture from drying during manipulation.

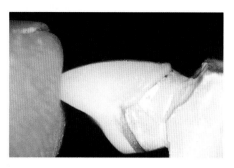

Fig 6-7o

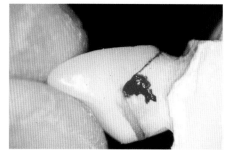

Fig 6-7p

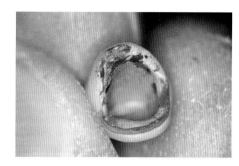

Fig 6-7q

Fig 6-7o Restoration with margin addition, seated onto die. After lubricating the die and removing any porcelain found inside the casting, the restoration is placed onto the die and pressed firmly until completely seated. This can be verified by examining the lingual metal margin. Slight vibration with a serrated instrument may be necessary to accomplish this.

Fig 6-7p After a separate firing, the restoration is reseated. The shoulder of the die is coated with an indicator to show high spots that prevent complete seating.

Fig 6-7q Red indicator shows area of the margin that prevents restoration from seating completely. These spots are very carefully removed with a worn diamond point. The restoration might have to be reseated several times before all high spots are removed. A microscope should be used to recognize a perfect seal.

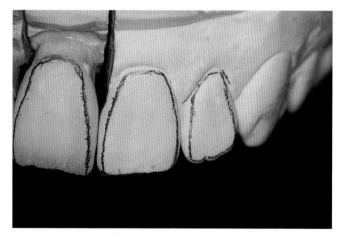

Fig 6-7r Seated restoration on master working model. Once the porcelain margins have been finalized, the restorations are placed back onto the working model and contoured. The remaining natural dentition is used as a guide for basic contour. To obtain a glaze, the restoration should be hand polished rather than fired.

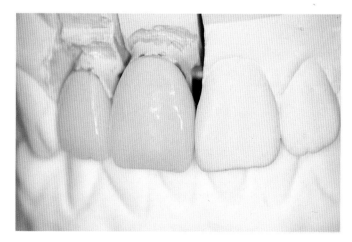

Fig 6-7s Glazed restorations. Hand polishing was used rather than furnace glaze, which could cause the porcelain margin to shrink and result in an open labial margin. The restorations are articulated. Lateral excursions and protrusive movement are performed to ensure proper function.

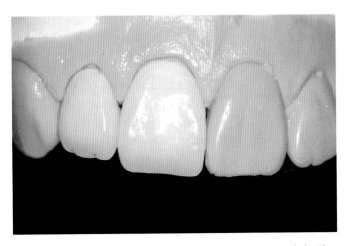

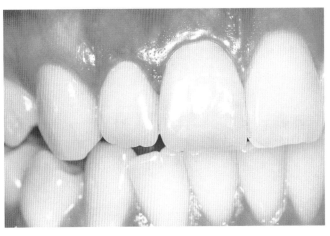

Fig 6-7t Completed restorations on tissue model. The tissue model is used throughout the entire procedure: waxing stage, metal substructure, and finished restoration. The tissue model was especially important in this case because defects in the gingiva were the main reason for restoring these teeth.

Fig 6-7u Seated maxillary right central and lateral incisor restorations after 3-day patient recall. Note how well the gingiva has adapted to the well-glazed porcelain margin. Left lateral excursion reveals no need for incisal adjustment. Proper use of a reliable articulator during fabrication will ensure an adjustment-free restoration after seating. This is important to the dentist and to ensure an esthetic result.

Fig 6-7v Seated maxillary right central and lateral incisor restorations in protrusive position with no necessary adjustments. Note the contour and color harmony the restorations have with the natural dentition (ie, line angles, incisal edge position and contour, labial texture and glaze, and CTC using the no-maverick method for duplication). Thorough case planning ensures a successful restoration.

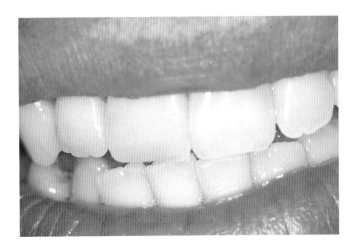

Case 8: Replacing Two Missing Maxillary Lateral Incisors (Figs 6-8a to o)

Description and Evaluation

A 35-year-old woman neglected oral hygiene and was in need of cosmetic improvement. Missing maxillary lateral incisors allowed the central incisors and canines to drift.

Goals and Concerns

1. Restore anterior teeth with two 3-unit splints, replacing two maxillary lateral incisors.
2. Fabricate provisional splint with functional and esthetic needs that will eventually be incorporated into the permanent restoration.
3. Construct anterior index of mounted provisional splint, which will be used throughout the fabrication of the permanent restoration.
4. Construct anterior guide table.
5. Duplicate CTC.
6. Establish centric stops and glide path developed with excursions and protrusive movement.

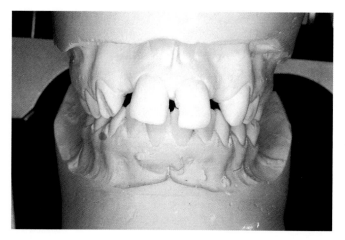

Fig 6-8a Articulated diagnostic model of patient's maxillary arch showing the extent of her poor oral maintenance. Model shows missing lateral incisors and drifting central incisors. An articulated diagnostic model should accompany every case sent to the laboratory. This is especially important if the laboratory is separate from the office and where there is no personal contact between the dentist and technician. Most technicians do not have the opportunity to see the patient; the articulated diagnostic model is the next best thing. It shows the laboratory the functional and esthetic needs of the patient (ie, premature contacts, lateral interferences, anterior guidance, anterior tooth length and contour, group function and posterior disocclusion).

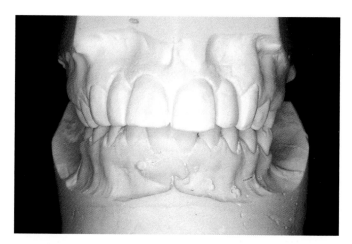

Fig 6-8b Articulated model of seated provisional restoration with incorporated functional needs. The provisional restoration is constructed by using the diagnostic model as a starting point and waxing missing teeth to it, as in this case, or by waxing an entirely new restoration after the teeth have been prepared. Functional needs are incorporated into both methods. In the former, esthetic improvements are not as pronounced as in the latter, with the understanding that the esthetic improvements will be made during fabrication of the permanent restoration. The latter method provides the laboratory with more information about the esthetic needs.

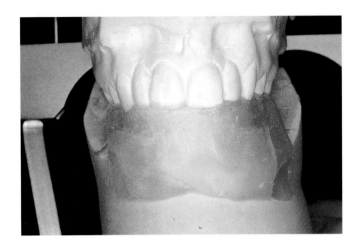

Fig 6-8c Articulated model of seated provisional restoration with wax anterior index. The anterior index can be constructed with flexible material (eg, silicone or rubber-base material) or firm materials (eg, stone or hard wax). The anterior index dictates the incisal edge position and contour of the permanent restoration. Once this has been established on the provisional restoration and duplicated in the model, it is transferred to the anterior index. Other than minor esthetic changes, the basic position and contour should be maintained. The index also dictates labial thickness of the restoration.

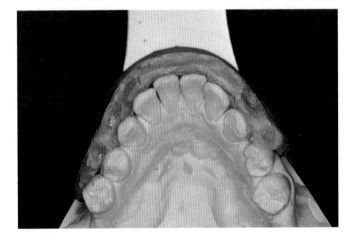

Fig 6-8d Anterior index showing incisal position and contour developed by the incisal edge of the provisional restoration. This should be used during the four stages of fabrication: waxing, metal preparation, porcelain buildup, and final contouring. The anterior index and anterior guide table will form the labial and lingual contours of the restoration. They must be used in conjunction with each other while making changes during each stage in order to satisfy both.

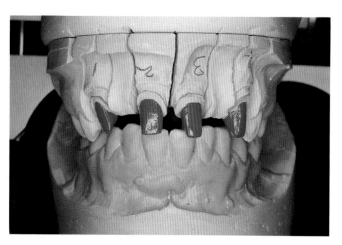

Fig 6-8e

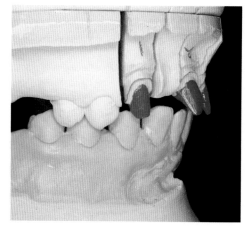

Fig 6-8f

Fig 6-8e Frontal view of mounted master working model ready for waxing. Die spacer has been applied over entire die except shoulder area. Also note maximum tooth reduction on the distal surfaces of the central incisors; it helps parallel the path of insertion and gives the technician an opportunity to improve on their shape by narrowing them while eliminating diastemata. This is a typical example of how important case planning is when attempting to obtain optimum contour in a restoration. The dentist must evaluate each case before preparation so that the laboratory has the best possible working conditions.

Fig 6-8f Lateral view of mounted master working model showing anterior maxillary and mandibular tooth relationship. Note angulation (splaying of the central incisors) and the potential problem with the path of insertion. For this reason, it was decided during case planning to fabricate two 3-unit bridges with detachment between the central incisors. Other potential problems include establishing ideal contour and color, due to the position of the incisal third. Close evaluation of the mounted master working model must be made before waxing begins.

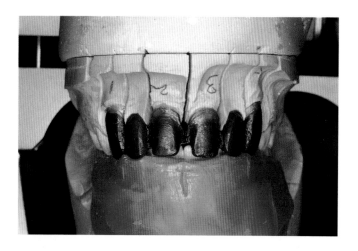

Fig 6-8g Wax patterns ready for investing. The restorations are waxed to full contour using the anterior matrix as a guide for incisal position and basic labial contour. Once this has been completed the wax patterns are cut back, leaving adequate room for porcelain. Note the red die spacer showing through the wax on the labial surface of the central incisors. This indicates a very thin casting (due to tooth splaying), which is necessary for obtaining sufficient room for porcelain. For thin castings such as this, a semiprecious or nonprecious alloy should be considered. Their superior strength surpasses that of noble alloys.

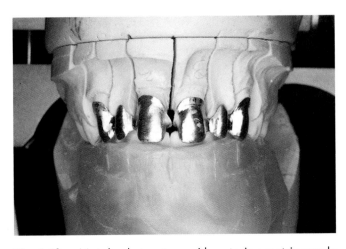

Fig 6-8h Metal substructure with anterior matrix ready for opaque application. A semiprecious (6% gold) alloy was selected for this case because of the thin metal substructure. The castings are dressed down to conform to the anterior matrix, making sure the substructure will supply maximum support for porcelain coverage. If care is taken during the waxing stage, little metal work will be necessary. After the needs of the anterior matrix are fulfilled, excursions and protrusive movements are made to confirm proper function dictated by the anterior guide table.

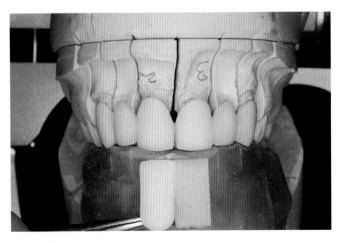

Fig 6-8i Fired dentin is compared to the hue-chroma and maverick CTC tabs (maverick plus hue-chroma duplicating method). The opaque layer corresponds to the hue-chroma dimension. The transition layer is a mixture of opaque and selected color dimensions for the CTC and is fired over the opaque. The dentin layer is then applied and fired, leaving room for a thin application of enamel porcelain. The customized tooth color tabs will determine at this time whether or not the fired dentin complies with the detected CTC. Any necessary color adjustments should be made before enamel application.

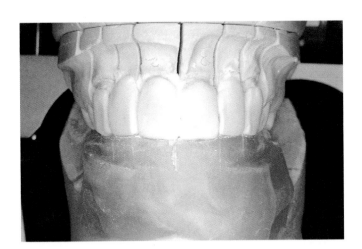

Fig 6-8j Prefired enamel application. If no color changes are needed after the dentin firing, enamel (value dimension) is applied to fill the anterior matrix completely. In most cases, the enamel layer is thin (much thinner than natural enamel) — thickest at the incisal edge and thinning toward the gingival third. Enamel porcelain is slightly overbuilt incisally to compensate for shrinkage.

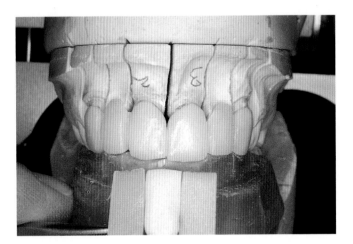

Fig 6-8k Three selected CTC tabs (value, hue-chroma, and maverick) are compared with the fired enamel. At this point the CTC should have been attained. Note the influence each tab has on the CTC. If the incisal edge was properly overbuilt, there should be little if any adjustments necessary to comply with the anterior index. The next step is to verify anterior guidance.

237

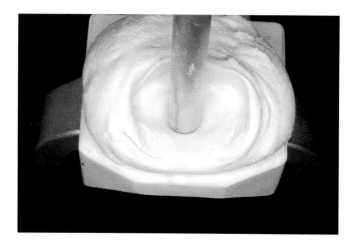

Fig 6-8l Customized anterior guide table. The working contour (any surface in contact with the tip of the incisal guide pin during articulator manipulation) of the customized anterior guide table represents all of the functional ingredients found in the provisional restoration. Note the high walls of the table, which indicate the steep incline the anterior teeth must take during anterior guidance. This information is transmitted to the restoration by forming its lingual contour.

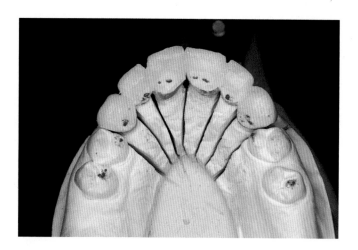

Fig 6-8m Lingual centric stops. Functional contour begins with establishing centric stops. This should begin during porcelain buildup; however, some contouring is usually necessary after firing. A centric stop should have a definite seat and should never be located on an incline. The red spots are lightly ground, giving way to a small flat surface.

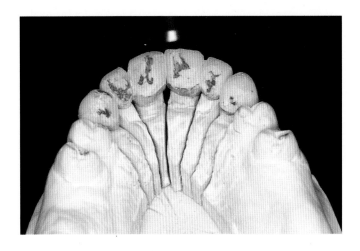

Fig 6-8n Tentative glide paths (red marking) made during excursive and protrusive movements. The red marking will be gradually ground away until a smooth glide path is established while maneuvering the guide pin over the surface of the customized anterior guide table. Eventually the exact contour of the guide table will be transferred to the lingual surface of the restoration as the incisal edge of the mandibular anterior teeth glide over it. This ensures the preservation of functional and phonetic qualities of the provisional restoration.

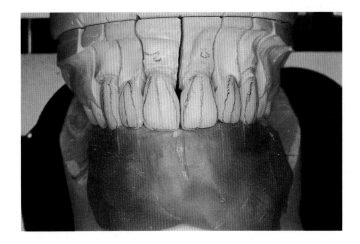

Fig 6-8o Contoured restorations ready for glaze. The restoration is brought to this point with the combined efforts of the diagnostic model, CTC guide, provisional restoration, anterior index, and customized anterior guide table. Note line angles and long axis that form basic contour of the restored teeth and the esthetic improvement over the provisional restoration (see Figs 6-8b and c). This is a typical example of how planning can help in the fabrication of a restoration, restoring function, contour, and color. The results should be the same, whether the laboratory is in the office or not.

Case 9: Replacing Missing Maxillary Central Incisors With Ceramic Implants (Figs 6-9 a to m)

Description and Evaluation

An 18-year-old woman lost her maxillary left central incisor in an accident with extensive bone and tissue damage. The case presented several problems that created a challenge for fabrication and an acceptable esthetic restoration. A ceramic implant with tissue augmentation was preferred in lieu of a three-unit bridge.

Goals and Concerns

1. Treatment will include a ceramic implant and a porcelain-to-metal restoration with a porcelain margin.
2. Tissue augmentation will be performed after the restoration is seated permanently.
3. CTC must be selected from an unprepared maxillary right central incisor.
4. Possible contour problem due to crown length and angulation of the implant.

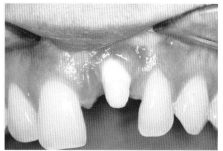

Fig 6-9a

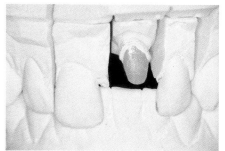

Fig 6-9b

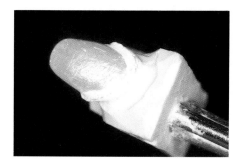

Fig 6-9c

Fig 6-9a Ceramic implant in place and prepared to accept a porcelain-to-metal restoration with porcelain margin. Note implant position and tissue damage that will lead to a potential esthetic problem. Missing maxillary left central incisor made it necessary to use the right central incisor for shade selection. Even with this unprepared tooth it is obvious that the maverick dimension is not present. Therefore the most appropriate method for tooth color duplication is the no-maverick method, where only two color dimensions are of concern: hue-chroma and value.

Fig 6-9b Articulated master working model with spacer die. Note steep overbite that could create a functional problem. The restoration must be designed to accept only a minimum load during excursions and protrusive movement. In cases where there are functional maxillary anterior teeth, a customized anterior guide table is not necessary. The canines work during left and right excursions, while the incisors work during protrusive movement.

Fig 6-9c Die of ceramic implant, which was prepared for a porcelain margin. It is important that a ceramic implant not be overprepared. There must be sufficient thickness for strength. For this reason, only the labial surface is prepared with a shoulder to accept the porcelain margin; the lingual surface is feather-edged to accept a metal margin.

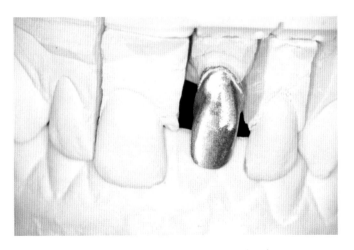

Fig 6-9d Semiprecious casting ready for opaque. Semiprecious alloy (6% gold) was used for needed strength. Note shape and length of the casting for optimum porcelain support. Casting is sprayed with 50-μm-alumina oxide then rinsed with either steam or ultrasonic cleaner (distilled water). Casting should be dried with a clean tissue or towel, never with compressed air, which is often contaminated with oil and/or foreign particles.

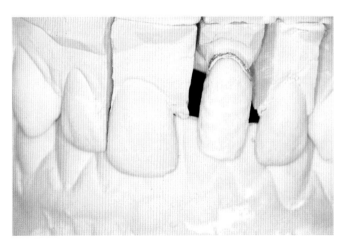

Fig 6-9e Casting with transition layer. Composite tooth color should be evaluated at this stage with the customized tooth color tabs used to measure the color dimensions at the time of tooth preparation. Selected color dimensions should be evident at this stage (compare to Fig 6-9a). Any noticeable discrepancy should be corrected before the dentin layer is applied. Note rough surface of the transition layer and the free margin at the shoulder of the die. Dentin porcelain will eventually be applied to this area.

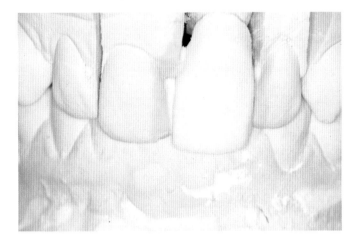

Fig 6-9f A layer of dentin porcelain (hue-chroma dimension) is applied over the transition layer and extended to the shoulder. A thin layer of enamel porcelain (value dimension) covers the dentin layer completely. Each layer can be fired separately or both can be fired together. Note overbuilt enamel at incisal edge to compensate for shrinkage.

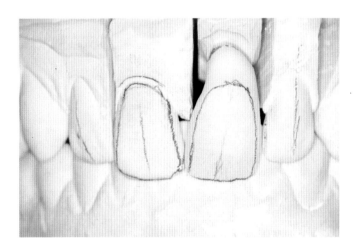

Fig 6-9g Labial contour. Porcelain buildup is fired and contoured. Labial contour is patterned after right central incisor. Note mesial and distal line angles and long axis. The gingival contour for the restoration is dictated by the tissue model. When surface texture is observed it should be included on the surface of the restoration.

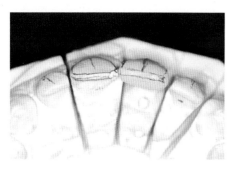

Fig 6-9h

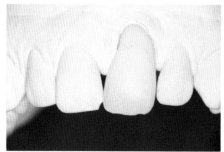

Fig 6-9i

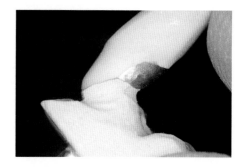

Fig 6-9j

Fig 6-9h Incisal edge position and contour. Like the labial surface, the position of the incisal edge is copied from the right central incisor. Terminal protrusive movement dictates its contour. During fabrication, porcelain should be built to the confines of the anterior matrix so only minor adjustments will be necessary during final contouring. It is also important to establish centric stop only, with no contact during excursions or protrusive movement (except terminal protrusive position).

Fig 6-9i Restoration on stone tissue model. The tissue model is used throughout the entire fabrication to ensure proper contour. This is especially important in cases with extensive tissue damage. A solid stone tissue model was used instead of a flexible silicone model so that mesial and distal contacts could be established. Uncut stone models can be used for showing tissue location as well as precise mesial and distal contacts.

Fig 6-9j Restoration seated on die, ready for glaze. Note angulation and lingual gingival contour of metal collar, which was shaped to satisfy the tissue model. The margin area was made thin and deep so as not to impinge on the tissue. There was insufficient room for porcelain coverage, thus a thin metal band was required. Note complete marginal seal, labially with porcelain, lingually with metal. This eliminates the possibility of roughness in this area and possible tissue irritation.

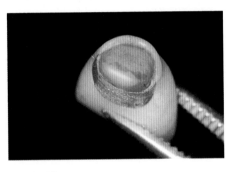

Fig 6-9k

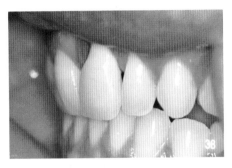

Fig 6-9l

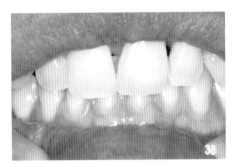

Fig 6-9m

Fig 6-9k Completed labial porcelain margin established using the dentin-to-shoulder method. The restoration is ready for glazing. If the seal is acceptable under microscopic observation, the restoration is hand polished. This is preferred over furnace glazing, which could cause slight porcelain distortions and result in an open margin. However, if there is an opening at the margin in the preglaze stage, a furnace glaze is required to fill this space and establish a perfect seal (firing temperature is approximately 5° to 7° below maturing temperature of dentin to prevent shrinkage).

Fig 6-9l Distal view of maxillary left central incisor restoration with porcelain-to-metal over a ceramic implant. Note contour at gingival third of restoration to accommodate future tissue augmentation. Note incisal edge position in accordance with that of the right central incisor and how well the tissue has adapted to the porcelain margin at the 3-day recall.

Fig 6-9m Labial view of seated restoration. Note mesial and distal contour and space left for eventual tissue augmentation, which is usually performed before restoration (patient preferred reverse procedure). Note mesial and distal contacts for support and very delicate labial texture, which conforms with that of the right central incisor. Hand polishing, as opposed to furnace glaze, helps preserve this texture as well as the porcelain margin. It is placed into the furnace, however, and fired to approximately 30° below maturing temperature of dentin to "semiglaze" before hand polishing.

Case 10: Replacing Missing Maxillary Right Central Incisor With a Cantilever Bridge (Figs 6-10a to n)

Description and Evaluation

A 45-year-old woman with missing maxillary right central incisor and devitalized left central incisor in need of a fixed appliance that will restore both teeth. Treatment plan included a post and core for the left central incisor and a porcelain-to-metal restoration. The patient requested that the restoration be as conservative as possible.

Goals and Concerns

1. Devitalized left central incisor was prepared to accept a post and core.
2. Porcelain-to-metal restoration will consist of a two-unit cantilever bridge with a rest on the right lateral incisor.
3. Porcelain margin will be included in the left central incisor restoration.
4. Impossible to use devitalized left central incisor for selecting CTC for the restoration; an unprepared tooth must serve this purpose.
5. Overall tooth color is not in the normal tooth color range. The maverick and enamel method for CTC duplication will be used.

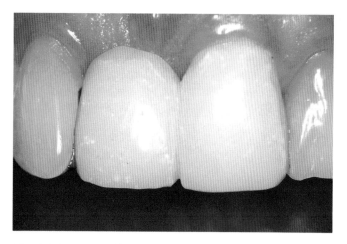

Fig 6-10a Maxillary provisional restoration worn by the patient during treatment. A model of this will provide the laboratory with the basic functional and esthetic needs of the patient. (The post and core has not been seated at this stage; it will be constructed with the porcelain restoration.)

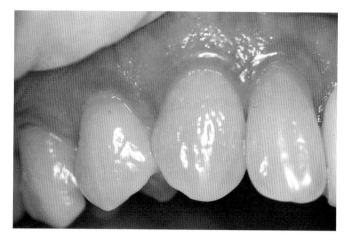

Fig 6-10b Maxillary right quadrant that will be used to select the CTC for the permanent restoration. The ideal location for detecting and measuring the four tooth color dimensions is the semiprepared or fully prepared tooth where the dentin is visible. When this is not possible, as in this case where the tooth to be restored is not vital, an unprepared tooth must be used. The right quadrant was used for this purpose. (Note different concentrations of the same family color from tooth to tooth.)

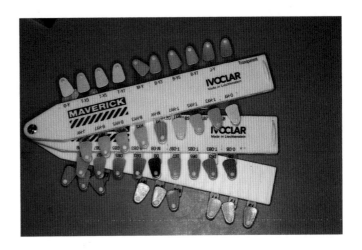

Fig 6-10c Maverick color guide. This color guide was designed to measure the maverick color dimension of the CTC. The color guide consists of tabs in four basic family colors (yellow, honey yellow, light brown, and dark brown) with dilutions along with opaque, transition, and enamel porcelains for each. In this case, where just two color dimensions are involved (maverick and value), the color guide will be used to select the dentin color and enamel.

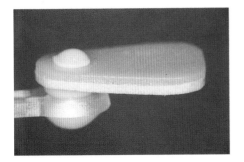

Fig 6-10d

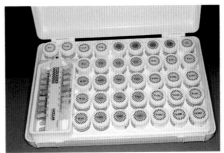

Fig 6-10e

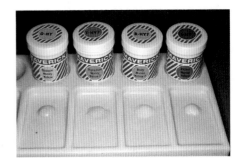

Fig 6-10f

Fig 6-10d Maverick color tab selected for the CTC of this case (honey yellow — 7). The color tab is made up of a layer of transition porcelain covered with dentin (body modifier). This tab would normally represent the dentin color of the prepared tooth. However, in this case it was used to compare with the maxillary right canine (see Fig 6-10b). Even though the canine is unprepared, this tab is more accurate than a commercial shade guide because the porcelains on the tab are those found in the Maverick Porcelain System (Ivoclar).

Fig 6-10e Maverick Porcelain System with customized tooth color guide. This system is used primarily for the maverick and enamel method for duplication. When the dentin has darkened to the degree that it is out of the range of the hue-chroma color dimension, the Maverick Porcelain System is used to satisfy needed CTC duplication. With the four available color families in the system, individual or combined, any color found in the natural dentition can be duplicated.

Fig 6-10f The four porcelains that will be used to duplicate the CTC for the restoration (HY-7). The porcelains will be applied in layers, and each layer will have a certain effect in the duplicating process: the opaque covers the metal substructure, blocking out any influence it might have on the composite color; the transition layer is a buffer zone between the opaque and dentin; the dentin layer (body buildup) corresponds to the dentin color of the tooth; and the enamel covers the restoration completely.

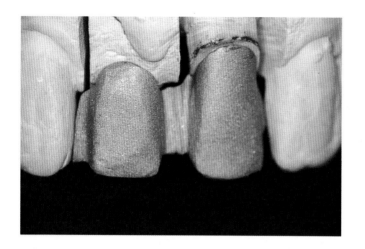

Fig 6-10g Metal substructure for the restoration. The substructure was waxed to full contour then cut back to leave space for an even amount of porcelain over the entire restoration. Both units were contoured to give maximum support for the porcelain. Note sturdy interproximal connection and shoulder of the die left free for porcelain. The pontic was extended to contact the tissue so that only a minimum thickness of porcelain is required to complete its length; this increases compression strength. A distal rest was included in the pontic and contacted the lingual surface of the right lateral incisor.

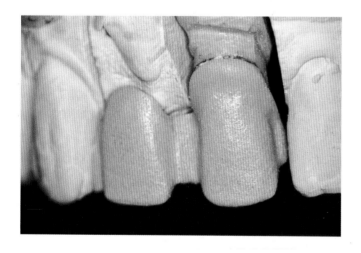

Fig 6-10h Opaque layer (O-HY) and porcelain margin. Premixed opaque that corresponds to dentin color (see Fig 6-10d) is fired to maturing temperature, after which porcelain margin material is applied and fired at a somewhat lower maturing temperature. The opaque layer is the foundation color for the composite color and will influence it greatly. The porcelain margin material color should be compatible with that of the dentin. A second margin application and firing were required to compensate for shrinkage.

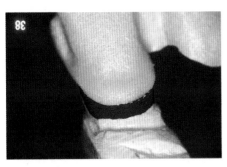

Fig 6-10i

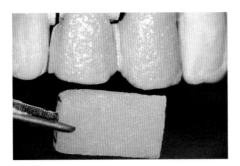

Fig 6-10j

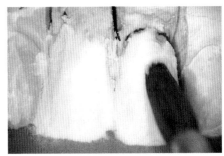

Fig 6-10k

Fig 6-10i Porcelain margin with red indicator. After the second margin application and firing, the restoration is seated onto the die with a red indicator that will show any "high spots" that might prevent the restoration from seating perfectly onto the die. If properly manipulated, only minor adjustments will be necessary. When the restoration is perfectly seated, the porcelain margin is tapered so dentin will cover it completely.

Fig 6-10j Fired transition layer with customized color tab (T-HY-7). The transition layer is a premixed porcelain made up of opacifiers and dentin and body modifiers that complement the composite color. The surface is roughened during application. Its purpose is to cancel the effects of the underlying opaque while contributing color needed for the composite effect. the rough surface helps diffuse light, which projects these colors in many directions. This porcelain layer is fired at a temperature approximately 10° lower than that of the porcelain margin material.

Fig 6-10k Body buildup (B-HY-7). Dentin is built to full contour minus the space needed for enamel. HY-7 is built within the confines of the anterior matrix and covers the transition layer completely. Any necessary internal modification should be incorporated during this application. The maturing temperature of this layer is approximately 10° lower than that of the transition layer because of its composition. Also, this lower maturing temperature ensures that the rough surface of the transition layer will remain.

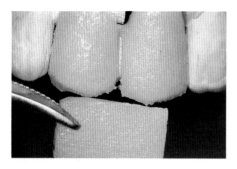

Fig 6-10l

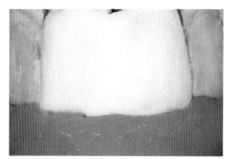

Fig 6-10m

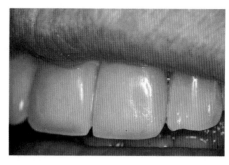

Fig 6-10n

Fig 6-10l Fired dentin layer compared to the CTC tab made up of a layer of transition material covered completely with dentin (HY-7). A customized color tab such as this can be used as well as one from the maverick color guide (see Fig 6-10d). The tab can be used after each firing, from the opaque layer to the enamel. (Note the surface of the transition layer has remained rough through the dentin firing.)

Fig 6-10m Prefired enamel application. Enamel covers the entire restoration, extending incisally to the anterior index (overbuilt slightly to compensate for shrinkage). Fine texturing is incorporated into this layer with a special brush after contour has been completed. The texture is retained after firing by hand polishing, eliminating a furnace glaze, which could destroy it.

Fig 6-10n Seated maxillary restoration. The restoration was conservative yet satisfied the functional and esthetic needs of the patient. The maverick and enamel duplicating method was used to obtain the CTC. The dentin color was out of the normal tooth color range. In cases such as this, color family is of prime importance; color concentration is secondary. A porcelain system with premixed porcelains is responsible for these results (see Fig 6-10e). The rest on the right central incisor pontic received support for the restoration from the right lateral incisor. Contour was patterned after maxillary lateral incisors.

Case 11: Correcting Occlusion With Maxillary and Mandibular Restorations (Figs 6-11a to o)

Description and Evaluation

This 55-year-old patient was in need of maxillary and mandibular restorations. Most of the problem was due to malocclusion and neglect, which caused tooth and periodontal breakdown. During case planning, it was decided to replace the missing teeth with double-abutted bridges while attempting to improve function to help retain the remaining dentition.

Goals and Concerns

1. Correct occlusion with properly contoured restorations.
2. The CTC is out of hue-chroma color range; must use maverick and enamel method for CTC duplication.
3. Two different color families recognized during CTC detection.
4. Irregularities will be incorporated internally with stains and modifiers.
5. Impossible to obtain natural contour of left central incisor due to incisal edge position and contour of mandibular anterior teeth.

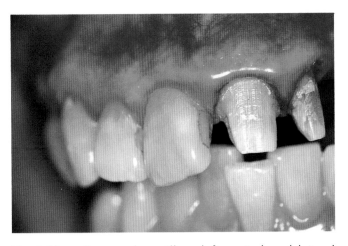

Fig 6-11a Prepared maxillary left central and lateral incisors that will act as anterior double abutments for a six-unit bridge. Note malocclusion (mandibular anterior teeth) that helped cause damage to these teeth. Color dimension detection indicates that the dentin is out of the hue-chroma color range, thus making it imperative that the maverick and enamel duplicating method be used to develop CTC.

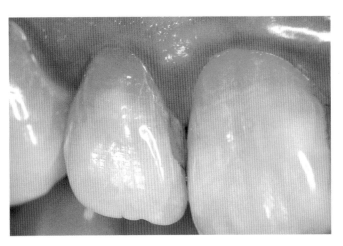

Fig 6-11b Maxillary right lateral and central incisors. Unprepared teeth reveal two different color families when comparing the lateral and central incisors. This is unusual and should be considered in the restoration.

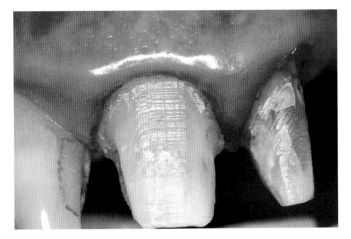

Fig 6-11c Prepared central and lateral incisors. Detection and measurement of tooth color dimensions verify the difference in color families as found in unprepared teeth (see Fig 6-11b). The central incisor was found to be in the light brown color family (LB-3), the lateral dark brown (DB-3), determined by a customized tooth color guide. The matching tab denotes the parts of neutral porcelain (three) that must be mixed with one part of light brown and dark brown body modifier, respectively, to comply with the CTC of the restoration.

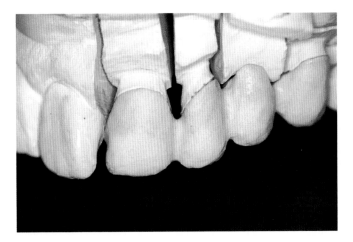

Fig 6-11d Fired opaque layer of maxillary restoration. The opaque layer forms the color foundation for the CTC. When the maverick dimension is the sole color source of the CTC, the opaque must be hand mixed to complement the CTC or it should be mixed from a porcelain system made especially to meet these needs (eg, Williams Dental Company).

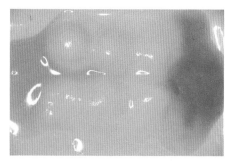

Fig 6-11e

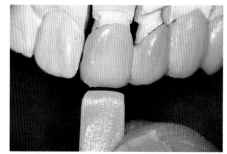

Fig 6-11f

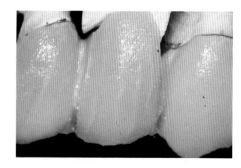

Fig 6-11g

Fig 6-11e   A mixture formulated to comply with the CTC of the restoration. The mixture consists of one part light brown body modifier, one part dark brown body modifier, and three parts neutral porcelain for each. This will be applied over the transition layer and could be described as the body buildup (dentin). The mixture is separated, dark brown for the lateral incisor and light brown for the central incisor, canine, and posterior teeth.

Fig 6-11f   Fired dentin is compared with customized color tab selected for the restored central incisor (LB-3). Irregularities are incorporated during this stage of fabrication. Their effects will be transmitted through a thin enamel layer. Note the color family difference between the lateral and central incisors (see Fig 6-11c).

Fig 6-11g   Close-up view of dentin layer with craze and check lines (lateral incisor and canine pontic). Interproximal areas are sliced with a thin blade before firing to allow each unit to shrink uniformly. This promotes more accurate color, stronger porcelain, and the opportunity to incorporate controlled interproximal color deposits found in the unprepared maxillary right central and lateral incisors and canine (see Fig 6-11a).

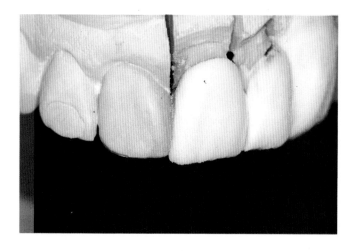

Fig 6-11h   Thin layer of prefired enamel porcelain overbuilt to compensate for shrinkage. Contouring during this stage, with the help of the anterior guide table, is important so that final functional contouring will be minimal. The enamel (value dimension) regulates the brightness of the underlying dentin (maverick dimension).

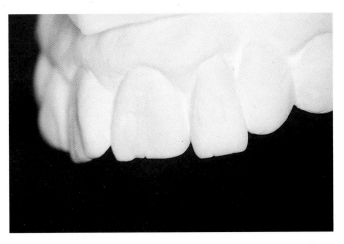

Fig 6-11i Pretreatment diagnostic model of maxillary arch. Note deformed left central incisor and extruded lateral incisor brought about by malocclusion. A treatment plan is established to correct problems that are often visible on the diagnostic model after corrections have been made. The diagnostic model, as in this case, often cannot be changed because of the opposing dentition. Therefore, the left central incisor restoration will have to be patterned somewhat after the original tooth. A diagnostic model should accompany every case sent to the laboratory.

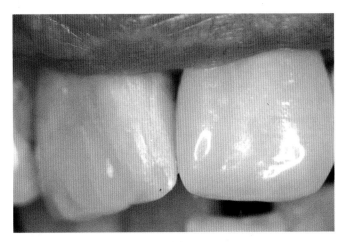

Fig 6-11j Seated maxillary restoration. Precise final contouring for this case was essential for its success due to the complicated occlusion. Note contour of left central incisor restoration as compared to the right. The incisal edge of the mandibular anterior teeth dictated this contour during left and right lateral excursions and posterior movement (rounded distal incisal edges). Minor adjustment to opposing dentition has made possible slight improvement over the diagnostic model. Note how well the composite color compares with the right central incisor (maverick and enamel duplicating method).

Fig 6-11k Prepared mandibular right canine and first premolar for five-unit bridge. Dentin revealed same color family and concentration as maxillary left central incisor, LB-3 (see Fig 6-11c). Note short premolar caused by occlusal wear and lack of room occlusally for the restoration. During case planning it must be decided which material will cover the occlusal surface: porcelain, porcelain-metal combination, or full-metal coverage. Available occlusal space is a prime determinant. It was decided to use porcelain occlusal.

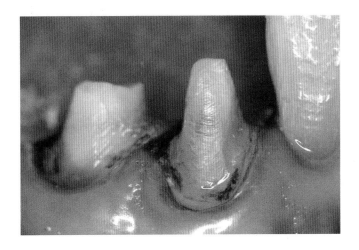

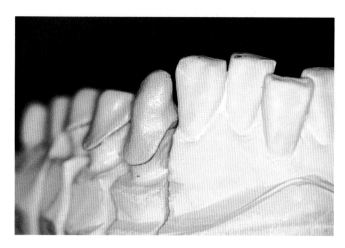

Fig 6-11l Opaque layer of mandibular restoration. Spray opaquing has a definite advantage over hand-applied opaque, especially in cases where space is at a premium. Color modifications are brushed in after the initial spray application. The opaque layer must complement the transition layer in order to accomplish the correct composite color for the restoration.

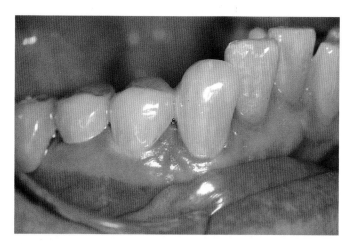

Fig 6-11m Seated mandibular restoration. The transition layer, dentin, and enamel were applied and fired as in the maxillary restoration. Irregularities were incorporated into the dentin. Combined thickness of metal, opaque, transition layer, dentin, and enamel measures approximately 3/4 mm (compare to Fig 6-11k). Occlusal surface had sufficient room for minimum porcelain coverage to fulfill required functional requirements (cusp tip-to-fossa occlusion).

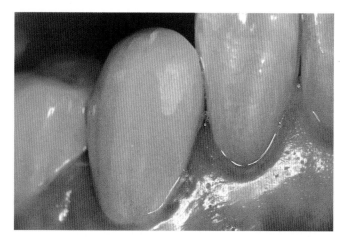

Fig 6-11n Magnified view of restored abnormally contoured mandibular right canine. Malocclusion and functional movements dictated its incisal edge position and contour. Ideal contour would have interfered with incisal functional needs of the patient. Note how well the composite color of the restoration compares with the natural right lateral incisor, in spite of thin porcelain. Accurate color detection and measurement were responsible for this.

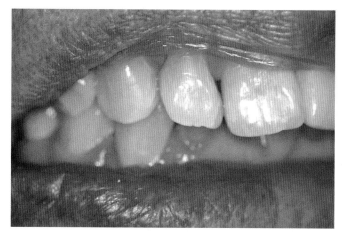

Fig 6-11o Mandibular restoration occluding with maxillary arch. The patient's malocclusion is quite obvious, as is the reason for the abnormally contoured mandibular right canine. Maxillary and mandibular restorations helped correct the problem to a certain extent in that they prevented further damage to the remaining natural dentition. Had the patient sought help sooner, a more positive prognosis could have been made.

Summary

Every case, regardless how simple, should be planned. Case planning should involve the dentist and technician and, whenever feasible, the patient. Today, patients are more concerned about cosmetic improvement and expect flawless results. Their comments and expectations should be aired during case planning to help the dentist decide the most appropriate treatment plan. It is not always possible to fulfill all the expectations of the patient, but when selecting a treatment plan that favors these expectations, the patient is usually more satisfied with the final restoration.

Index